*Six Steps to Managing
Alzheimer's Disease and Dementia*

Six Steps to Managing Alzheimer's Disease and Dementia

A Guide for Families

ANDREW E. BUDSON, MD
Neurology Service, Section of Cognitive & Behavioral Neurology, &
Center for Translational Cognitive Neuroscience,
Veterans Affairs Boston Healthcare System
Alzheimer's Disease Research Center & Department of Neurology,
Boston University School of Medicine
Division of Cognitive & Behavioral Neurology, Department of Neurology,
Brigham and Women's Hospital
Harvard Medical School
Boston, MA
Boston Center for Memory
Newton, MA

MAUREEN K. O'CONNOR, PSYD
Psychology Service, Section of Neuropsychology,
Bedford Veterans Affairs Hospital
Bedford, MA
Alzheimer's Disease Research Center & Department of Neurology,
Boston University School of Medicine
Boston, MA

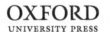

OXFORD
UNIVERSITY PRESS

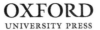

OXFORD

UNIVERSITY PRESS

Oxford University Press is a department of the University of Oxford. It furthers
the University's objective of excellence in research, scholarship, and education
by publishing worldwide. Oxford is a registered trade mark of Oxford University
Press in the UK and certain other countries.

Published in the United States of America by Oxford University Press
198 Madison Avenue, New York, NY 10016, United States of America.

Library of Congress Cataloging-in-Publication Data
Names: Budson, Andrew E., author. | O'Connor, Maureen K., author.
Title: Six steps to managing Alzheimer's disease and dementia : a guide for
families / Andrew E. Budson, M.D., and Maureen K. O'Connor, PsyD
Description: New York, NY : Oxford University Press, [2022] |
Includes bibliographical references and index.
Identifiers: LCCN 2020048282 (print) | LCCN 2020048283 (ebook) |
ISBN 9780190098124 (hardback) | ISBN 9780190099909
Subjects: LCSH: Alzheimer's disease—Treatment. | Dementia—Treatment.
Classification: LCC RC523.S59 2021 (print) | LCC RC523 (ebook) |
DDC 616.8/311—dc23
LC record available at https://lccn.loc.gov/2020048282
LC ebook record available at https://lccn.loc.gov/2020048283

DOI: 10.1093/med/9780190098124.001.0001

3 5 7 9 8 6 4 2

Printed by Integrated Books International, United States of America

Contents

Preface

"I always thought I had a lot of patience, but if he asks me what we are doing today one more time, I think I will scream."

"I love my wife but I have no time for myself—I haven't been able to go to the gym or visit my friends or even see my doctor."

"He wants to drive but I don't know if it's safe."

"I've never fooled around in my life and now, at age 83, my wife is accusing me of having an affair."

"It's happening every evening now—she keeps saying that she needs to go 'home,' but we already are home."

"He won't use his walker and I'm afraid he's going to fall."

"I don't mind cleaning up when she doesn't make it to the bathroom, but now she's fighting me when I try to get her washed up."

"When I came home from the hairdresser he asked me who I was—he really didn't recognize me."

"Yesterday I found a pan burning on the stove, so now I can't leave her alone anymore."

Do some of these experiences sound familiar?

Do you find that just when you've solved one problem, another problem pops up and you're back to square one?

Do you feel that no one could possibly cope with all the problems you're dealing with?

Do you find it frustrating that no one really understands what you're going through?

Is your own health beginning to suffer?

Do you want to understand what causes dementia and how to manage all the issues that go with it?

Are you worried that some of the medications being given are actually making things worse?

Would you like to learn what medications can be used to make things better?

Would you like to learn new ways to sustain your relationship with your loved one?

Are you feeling so tired that sometimes you wish it could all just be over?

If you answered "yes" to any of these questions, this book was written for you. We can help you. Caring for someone with Alzheimer's disease or another dementia can be one of the most frustrating, exhausting, and heartbreaking activities that one can do—but it can also be fulfilling and rewarding. We will show you how to be a better care partner and caregiver. In these pages we explain why different problems and behaviors arise, and how to manage them when they do. We review which medications are helpful—and which are likely to make things worse. We explain how to care for yourself, and why that is so important for both you and your loved one. We can show you how to sustain your relationship with your loved one and how to plan for the future.

In our practices as a neurologist and a neuropsychologist, we have worked with several thousand families who are struggling with dementia, just like you. We give them tips for communication to diffuse tense situations. We explain why their loved ones may have false memories, hallucinate, not recognize them, or think they have been replaced by an imposter. We also help them deal with tremors, falls, wandering, agitation,

aggression, and incontinence. This book provides us with the opportunity to tell you about these and other topics, in six straightforward steps.

Lastly, some of you might wonder how this book differs from our prior one, *Seven Steps to Managing Your Memory: What's Normal, What's Not, and What to Do About It*. In a very real sense, this book is the sequel to that one. *Seven Steps to Managing Your Memory* focuses on the older individual who is concerned about minor memory problems and either is aging normally, has mild cognitive impairment, or has just the very beginnings of Alzheimer's disease or another dementia. It discusses in great detail how to distinguish the changes in normal aging from those of Alzheimer's disease, what the doctor should do for the evaluation, what treatments are available for mild memory problems (as well as the depression and anxiety that often accompany them), how to optimize brain health with diet and exercise, and how to strengthen memory with activities, attitudes, strategies, and aids. In brief, *Seven Steps to Managing Your Memory* is written for the individual with mild memory problems. By contrast, this book is written for the families of individuals whose dementia has progressed beyond the mild stages and for those families who know things are heading in that direction and want to start planning for the future now.

Acknowledgments

The genesis of this book began with the excellent questions posed by the families of individuals with Alzheimer's disease and other causes of dementia. We thank them for the inspiration and guidance they have given us. We also thank our friends and family members who read various drafts of this book and provided their invaluable feedback: George Null, Richard Budson, Sandra Budson, Burt Shnitzler, Judy Bergman, Olga Quinlan, Pam Molnar, Eric Bender, Fred Dalzell, Peter Grinspoon, Ron Elliott, and Ceci McVey; we couldn't have done it without you. We are also grateful to our colleagues and mentors who have taught us so much about caring for individuals with dementia, including Paul Solomon, Elizabeth Vassey, Kate Turk, Ana Vives-Rodriguez, Chad Lane, Kirk Daffner, Dan Press, Chris Jagiello, David LaPorte, Michael Franzen, Keith Hawkins, Richard Delany, Patricia Boyle, Malissa Kraft, Lee Ashendorf, Helen Denison, and Edith Kaplan.

The content of this book has been derived from the patients whom the authors have seen in their private practices along with literature reviews conducted solely for the purpose of this book. These reviews and the writing of this book have been conducted during early mornings, late nights, weekends, and vacations. Their contribution to this book was conducted outside of both their VA tours of duty and their Boston University/ NIH research time.

Introduction

Caregiving is hard. It's hard whether you're caring for your spouse, parent, grandparent, sibling, other family member, or friend. Even if you had an extra 10 hours each day to do it, it's hard to manage all the problems that come with dementia. And caring for a loved one with dementia can sometimes feel like a long, lonely journey. That's one reason we've woven two stories into the book—to remind you that you are not alone. We hope that one of these stories will resonate with you. Let's consider the first story.

"Dad, where are you?" Sara asks into her phone. "Your neighbor called; she saw smoke coming out of your house. I'm here now. It looks like you left the stove on with something in the frying pan."

"Oh no, not again!" Jack exclaims. "I was trying to make an . . . make one of those things with eggs and cheese, but I didn't have any cheese. So I ran out to get some."

"OK, but you need to turn the stove off if you are leaving the house."

"I thought I turned it off—I've even got notes up to remind me—but I must have forgotten."

"Can you come home now? We need to clean things up."

"Well, that's another thing . . . I confess I was happy to see you calling me, because I'm sort of lost."

Sara takes in a deep breath as she thinks, *He used to know this city like the back of his hand.*

"OK, I just asked a guy," Jack continues. "He says I'm on Main Street near Panner Avenue, heading east."

"So, just make a U-turn; you'll be back in your neighborhood in 15 minutes."

"OK, great. Maybe you can stay on the phone in case I get lost."

Sara hears a grating and squeaking sound, followed by a loud pop.

"Dad, what was that noise! Are you alright?"

"Ah, Sara, I think I popped my tire. I guess I pulled too close to the curb."

"Just stay there, Dad," Sara says as she walks out of the house. "I'll come pick you up, and then we'll deal with your car."

Because he was diagnosed with both Alzheimer's disease and some small strokes 4 years ago, Sara understood that her father's memory was impaired and would get worse. She has been helping him to eat right, exercise, and use reminders to keep him healthy and independent. She's pleased with how well the two of them have worked together managing his memory problems and keeping him living on his own. With this latest episode, however, Sara is worried that her father won't be able to live at home much longer. She knows he's not ready for a nursing home, and they cannot afford a retirement community or assisted living. She wonders if he should move in with her and her daughter, but she's worried that it would create even more work for her. She doesn't know what to do.

Let's consider another story.

Martin has been managing Nina's dementia by himself. He's proud that he has been able to keep her at home.

"Hold on, honey, I'll be right there," Martin says as he looks at the clock. *3:15 AM.* He gets out of bed and catches up with Nina in the hallway.

"I know you were trying to make it to the bathroom," he says as he pulls off the wet nightgown and absorbent undergarment. "You just didn't make it in time, that's all. Not to worry."

He leads her into the bathroom and helps her sit down on the toilet. She's able to urinate a little more.

"OK," Martin says. "Let's get you cleaned up." He cleans her skin and helps her into a new undergarment and nightgown, then puts her back into their bed.

Martin is just starting to clean the hallway when she says, "I have to go."

"You just went, honey," he calls. "Try to go back to sleep."

"I have to go," she says again, sitting up in bed.

"Let's not go through this every night," he says, walking into the bedroom.

Martin then sees the urgent look in her eyes and suddenly understands. "OK, if you need to move your bowels, let's go."

But it is too late. Her undergarment, nightgown, and the bed linens are now soiled. He guides her into the bathroom again, wipes her a bit, and helps her sit down on the toilet. "Do you need to go anymore?"

She shakes her head no.

"Alright then," he says, smiling. "Let's get you cleaned up and back to bed. How about I give you a nice warm bath."

He runs the bathwater. With a little cajoling, she settles into the soapy water. "OK, you just relax in the tub for a minute while I clean up."

Fifteen minutes later she is in her third undergarment and nightgown and tucked into the clean sheets and blankets on the bed. Martin lies next to her, gently stroking her hair, until she falls asleep. Then he gets up and finishes cleaning the bedroom, hallway, and bathroom. Finally, he puts the dirty linens, towels, and nightgowns in the wash.

He looks at the clock as he crawls back into bed. *4:30 AM. Well, hopefully I'll get another hour of sleep*, he thinks as he closes his eyes.

Do the stories of either Sara and Jack or Martin and Nina sound familiar? We will be following these characters throughout the book to illustrate the six steps to managing Alzheimer's disease and dementia. We will be with them as we gain a better understanding of dementia (*Step 1*) and learn how to manage the problems that come with it (*Step 2*). We'll discover which medications can help—and which may actually make things worse (*Step 3*). We will see how they build their care team and learn to care for themselves (*Step 4*), in addition to sustaining their relationship with their loved one—despite the dementia (*Step 5*). Lastly, we will see how they plan for the future, the end, and beyond (*Step 6*).

We hope that these stories—composites of real families we have worked with—along with the guidance and other insights we'll be providing will make it easy to understand the issues you are facing and their implications. If, however, you would prefer to read the text without the stories, please do so. We've written the book so that the stories are optional.

Note that we try to be exhaustive in this book—discussing virtually every problem that could possibly arise. We certainly don't expect your loved one to have all or even half of these problems. But we want you to be prepared for them all.

Without further ado, we now turn to *Step 1* to understand what dementia is and how it is related to Alzheimer's disease.

Step 1

UNDERSTAND
DEMENTIA

Everyone is familiar with the terms "dementia" and "Alzheimer's disease," but not everyone knows exactly what they mean and how they are related. To begin our journey, we first need to develop a clear understanding of what dementia and Alzheimer's disease are.

1

What is dementia?

DEMENTIA MEANS PROBLEMS WITH THINKING AND MEMORY ARE IMPAIRING DAILY FUNCTION

Martin smiles as he thinks, *Good girl, Nina—you slept through the rest of the night.* It's only when he climbs out of bed that he realizes how tired he is.

"Good morning, Nina," he says as cheerfully as he can. "It's time to get up and get ready for your doctor's appointment."

She looks up at him with love as they shuffle off to use the bathroom. Then, hand over hand, he helps her brush her teeth. Back in their bedroom, he picks out clothes for her and guides her into them, starting with a disposable undergarment. Then he eases her into an armchair so that he can get himself ready.

When people have problems with their memory and thinking to the point that they can no longer function independently, they have dementia. People are diagnosed with dementia when three things are present:

1. Concern that there has been a prominent decline in thinking and memory by the individual, their family, or their doctor
2. Substantial impairment on formal tests of thinking and memory

3. The thinking and memory problems interfere with their everyday activities

DEMENTIA HAS DIFFERENT STAGES

Dementia is commonly divided into four stages:

- Very mild
- Mild
- Moderate
- Severe

Individuals with very mild dementia have difficulty doing one or two complex daily activities, such as doing housework, paying bills, preparing meals, shopping, or taking medicines, whereas those with mild dementia have trouble with most of these activities. Difficulties with one or two basic activities of daily living, such as dressing, bathing, eating, using the toilet, and controlling bowel and bladder, suggest that the dementia is in the moderate stage, whereas difficulties with most of these basic activities suggest that the severe stage is present. Each of these four stages lasts between approximately 1 to 4 years. The total time from a diagnosis of dementia in the very mild stage until death ranges from about 4 to 16 years, although it more commonly lasts 6 to 12 years.

DEMENTIA CAN BE CAUSED BY MANY DIFFERENT DISORDERS

Dementia is not a disease in itself; rather, it is a condition with many different causes. It is analogous to a headache. Headaches can be due to many different causes, such as muscle tension, migraines, a blood clot, or a tumor. Just like a headache, some causes of dementia are relatively benign and easily treatable, whereas other causes are more serious and may have no treatment. Alzheimer's is one disease that causes dementia. In fact, it is the cause of dementia between 60% and 70% of the time, which is why people often confuse Alzheimer's disease and dementia. Other common causes of dementia include vascular dementia, dementia with Lewy bodies, and frontotemporal dementia. We'll learn about the specific causes of dementia in *Chapters 2* and *3*.

PRIMARY CARE PROVIDERS MAY BE ABLE TO DETERMINE THE CAUSE OF DEMENTIA

Martin thinks about when it all started: Nina had trouble with her memory and complicated tasks. She might miss paying a bill or pay another one twice. She couldn't balance her checkbook. She had trouble with several computer programs that she had used for years.

Nina mentioned her memory difficulties to her doctor. The doctor spoke with both of them about her symptoms and ordered some blood work and an MRI scan of her brain. The nurse handed Martin a questionnaire to fill out while she gave Nina a 15-minute pencil-and-paper test of thinking and memory.

In straightforward cases, a primary care provider may be able to diagnose your loved one. The essential elements of any dementia evaluation include a review of the symptoms, blood work, pencil-and-paper tests of thinking and memory, and a brain scan (as described in the next paragraph). The doctor will typically begin by reviewing whether there are any difficulties with thinking, memory, language, behavior, incontinence, or walking, in addition to other relevant problems. Medications are reviewed as well to make sure none are impairing your loved one's memory, balance, or other functions (see *Chapter 12*). The examination of the blood includes basic tests to make sure there are no signs of infections or problems in

blood chemistry, in addition to special tests to rule out vitamin deficiencies and thyroid problems. Pencil-and-paper tests
of cognitive function are essential, because different patterns
of performance can suggest different disorders. In the primary
care setting, brief screening tests of thinking and memory are
typically used. These screening tests take 5 to 15 minutes and
often include remembering a few words, drawing a clock, and
doing simple arithmetic.

The basic brain imaging scans that may be recommended are
magnetic resonance imaging (more commonly known as MRI)
and computed tomography (more commonly known as CT or
"cat" scans). MRIs use a powerful magnet to look at the brain
and give better pictures than CT scans, which use X-rays, but
either test will show whether there is anything wrong with the
structure of the brain. An MRI or CT scan can detect brain disorders such as strokes, bleeds, tumors, fluid collections, multiple sclerosis, some infections, and many other disorders. You
can also see patterns of brain atrophy (shrinkage) that may be
common in one or another brain disease. However, patterns of
brain atrophy are just one piece of evidence that can be evaluated when the doctor is making a diagnosis. We cannot usually
know for sure that someone does or does not have a particular
brain disease just by looking at a brain imaging scan.

SCREENING TESTS MAY NOT BE ACCURATE FOR SOMEONE WHO IS HIGHLY EDUCATED, IS VERY BRIGHT, HAS A LEARNING DISABILITY, OR HAS A DIFFERENT CULTURAL BACKGROUND

Nina was surprised by the doctor's recommendation, exclaiming,
"The MRI and blood work didn't show any problems and I only
had a bit of trouble on the memory test, but you're sending me
to a memory center? Can't this just be normal aging?"

"It could be," the doctor explained. "But when someone is quite bright like you are—regardless of how much schooling they have had—a brief screening test like I gave you might not detect subtle thinking and memory problems. I want to send you to a neuropsychologist who can give you more challenging tests that will be able to determine whether these small declines in thinking and memory are part of normal aging or the beginning of dementia."

When interpreting tests of thinking and memory, we need to take into account intelligence as well as other factors, such as someone's culture, occupation, and any prior learning disabilities. Therefore, screening tests that can be performed quickly in a primary care setting are not the right tests for everyone. Sometimes the screening test will suggest that a memory disorder is present when, in actuality, the problem is a life-long learning disability or another factor. Screening tests can also miss small but very real signs of memory loss in someone who is extremely smart. In these cases, it is best to see a neuropsychologist or other memory specialist.

NEUROPSYCHOLOGISTS EVALUATE AND DIAGNOSE PROBLEMS WITH THINKING, MEMORY, AND BEHAVIOR

Neuropsychologists are psychologists who have received advanced training in the use and interpretation of pencil-and-paper tests and questionnaires to help diagnose brain disorders. Neuropsychological evaluations factor in how many years of education someone has, their age, cultural differences, prior learning disabilities, current or prior psychiatric disorders, and other factors that could impact an individual's performance on tests of thinking and memory. For most tests, instead of a simple "passing" or "failing" score, results are compared to those of other people who are the same age and have a similar background. For instance, a test result that is normal for an 80-year-old could represent a problem for someone age 50. Once they better understand the relative strengths and weaknesses of someone's thinking and memory, neuropsychologists also make specific recommendations of things that people can do to improve their function in daily life.

NEUROLOGISTS DIAGNOSE AND TREAT BRAIN DISORDERS

"Let me make sure I understand this," Nina said when she was told her diagnosis at the memory center. "You're saying that although my dementia is only mild, you think it's from two disorders—Alzheimer's plus dementia with Lewy bodies?"

"Yes," the neuropsychologist explained. "You had some trouble with the memory tests in a pattern that looks like Alzheimer's disease. Specifically, even when you learned information and could say it back to us, some of the information was rapidly forgotten. Rapid forgetting is common in Alzheimer's."

"OK, but what about this dementia with Lewy bodies?"

The neurologist leaned forward in his chair. "Do you remember telling me about seeing a dog or another animal in your bedroom on many nights? And Martin telling me about how you move around in your sleep—sometimes violently—as if you were acting out your dreams?"

"Yes. Is that how you know I have Lewy bodies?"

"That and the mild tremor in your hands, slight stiffness in your body, and your scuffing the floor a bit when you walk."

Neurologists are medical doctors who specialize in the diagnosis and treatment of disorders of the brain and other parts of the nervous system. When evaluating a patient for a memory disorder, they are on the lookout for anything that could be interfering with memory as they are going through a person's medical history, current medications, personal habits, lifestyle factors, family history, physical and neurological exam findings, blood work, and brain imaging studies. Note that although a straightforward memory evaluation does not require a neurologist or other specialist, if the evaluation is complicated or if a routine evaluation does not yield an answer, seeing a neuropsychologist, neurologist, psychiatrist, geriatrician, or other memory specialist can be helpful. Your loved one may be referred to one of these specialists by their primary care provider, or you may decide that you want to seek one of them out for a second opinion.

In addition to conducting the usual parts of a physical examination that most physicians do, a neurologist performs a specialized neurological exam to look for any problems with the brain or nervous system. This exam looks for problems such as strokes, tumors, Parkinson's disease, tremors, multiple sclerosis, and many other disorders that could be the cause of thinking and memory problems. Vision and hearing are always evaluated, because if one cannot see or hear well, it won't be possible to process, understand, and remember information coming in through the ears and eyes.

Not all neurologists specialize in memory disorders, so if your loved one is going to see a neurologist for their dementia, make sure the physician has been trained in or has experience with memory disorders. Psychiatrists and geriatricians are also physicians who may be trained in dementia; they may be the best specialist in your community for your loved one to see.

SUMMARY

Dementia is the term used to describe progressive impairment of thinking and memory that interferes with daily function. Dementia is not a specific disorder, it is a condition with many causes. Alzheimer's disease is the most common cause of dementia. Primary care providers are able to diagnose most straightforward cases of dementia, whereas specialists such as neuropsychologists, neurologists, psychiatrists, and geriatricians may be needed when the diagnosis is not straightforward. For a more detailed discussion of the evaluation of dementia and its possible causes, please see our book *Seven Steps to Managing Your Memory*.

Let's consider some examples to illustrate what we learned in this chapter.

- *You are concerned about your loved one's memory and you take them to see their doctor. The doctor diagnoses them with dementia. Should you be satisfied with that diagnosis?*
  ○ No! Dementia is not a disease in itself; it is a condition with many different causes. Go back to the doctor and ask what is the cause of the dementia. If they cannot give you an answer, you will need to take your loved one to a specialist.
- *Is dementia the same thing as Alzheimer's disease?*
  ○ No. Dementia is a general term indicating that thinking and memory have deteriorated to the point that daily function is impaired. Alzheimer's disease is one of many causes of dementia. Other causes of dementia include strokes, infections, vitamin deficiencies, and other neurological diseases.
- *I'm sure that my loved one has dementia, but I haven't taken them to see their doctor. Can the doctor actually do anything to help?*
  ○ Yes! Taking them to the doctor is very important. They may have an infection, vitamin deficiency, thyroid disorder, or depression such that, after treatment, their memory could improve—or even return to normal. In addition, in *Step 3* we will discuss medications available to help people with memory disorders that can make a real difference.

2

What is Alzheimer's disease?

Now that we understand what the term dementia means, we are ready to learn about the major neurological disorders that lead to dementia, beginning with Alzheimer's disease, the most common cause.

ALZHEIMER'S IS A BRAIN DISEASE CHARACTERIZED BY AMYLOID PLAQUES AND NEUROFIBRILLARY TANGLES

In 1906 a psychiatrist named Alois Alzheimer looked at brain tissue from one of his patients under a microscope and first saw these *amyloid plaques* and *neurofibrillary tangles*. We now know that the plaques are a mixture of a protein called beta amyloid, parts of brain cells, as well as other substances that are found between and outside the cells. Although we don't know exactly what the normal function of beta amyloid is, everyone's brain makes it. It may be involved in fighting off brain infections. Nevertheless, when too much beta amyloid accumulates, leading to plaques, Alzheimer's disease develops.

There is much research trying to understand the exact relationship between amyloid plaques and cognitive function. One explanation is as follows: When the plaques first form, they don't necessarily cause problems, but once the "cleanup cells" in the brain—part of the brain's immune system—begin to react to the plaques, an inflammatory reaction occurs that disrupts communication between brain cells and interferes with brain function.

Damage to the cells from the plaques causes neurofibrillary tangles to form inside them. We call them "tangles" because they look like tangled string under the microscope. The tangles are composed of tau, part of the skeleton and nutrient system of the dying brain cell (also called a neuron). Ultimately, as Alzheimer's disease progresses, more and more brain cells are damaged by plaques, form tangles, and die.

ALZHEIMER'S DISEASE HAS MANY STAGES

Sponge in hand, Sara is working with her father, Jack, to clean the soot from the kitchen after he left the stove on.

"Dad, do you know how many cans of corn you have in here?"

Jack joins Sara at the cupboard. "Holy moly! There must be 20 cans of corn in there!"

"Twenty-three. I counted them."

"Well, I guess I can't keep track of how many I have. I'll have to make a note not to buy any more corn. Now, where did I put that notebook . . ."

Sara moves on to clean the refrigerator.

"Dad, did you know you have spoiled food in here?"

"Do I? I guess I forgot about it."

Sara thinks about how her father's disease has progressed since he was diagnosed 4 years ago. *Well*, she sighs as she throws out something that might have been chicken a month ago, *his dementia has certainly gotten worse.*

Alzheimer's is a disease that starts in the brain years before any symptoms are noticeable. Over time, thinking and memory begin to be affected. When the deterioration in thinking and memory begin to cause problems with function, dementia is present.

In *very mild* Alzheimer's disease, function is impaired just a bit; for example, individuals may no longer be able to perform the complicated activities that they did previously, such as remodeling a bathroom or hosting a large dinner party. They have memory problems such that they often misplace things, and finding words may be difficult.

In *mild* Alzheimer's disease, forgetfulness and other problems with thinking begin to interfere with more routine activities such as cooking, shopping, and paying bills. Getting lost in familiar places and repeating questions and stories often become prominent, as new information is rapidly forgotten.

In *moderate* Alzheimer's disease, daily living activities, including dressing and bathing, become difficult. Learning new information may be impossible, word-finding problems are prominent, and changes in behavior and personality may occur.

In *severe* Alzheimer's disease, people have difficulty communicating, recognizing family members, and remaining continent.

ALZHEIMER'S DISEASE IS NOT PART OF NORMAL AGING

Given how common Alzheimer's disease is in individuals in their 70s and 80s, it is reasonable to wonder if Alzheimer's is just part of normal aging. However, there are many people who live into their 90s or even 100s without developing Alzheimer's disease either clinically or pathologically (when their brains are looked at after death under a microscope). In fact, it is estimated that roughly half of individuals age 85 and older do not have Alzheimer's or any other type of dementia. So, although Alzheimer's disease is more common with aging, it is not a normal part of it.

You may wonder if Alzheimer's disease is more common in women or in men. Of the 5.1 million people in the United States with Alzheimer's disease age 65 and older, approximately two-thirds are women. Why is that? Part of the answer is that Alzheimer's is more common as people age, and women live longer than men, but that may not be the only answer. Other explanations are being actively investigated.

FAMILY HISTORY OF ALZHEIMER'S DISEASE INCREASES THE CHANCES OF DEVELOPING IT

Because Alzheimer's is the most common disorder affecting thinking and memory in old age, we are all at risk for developing the disease, approaching 40% by age 85. If one has a family history of memory problems that sound like Alzheimer's disease in a parent or a sibling, the risk of Alzheimer's disease does rise, such that it becomes two to four times more likely that the memory problems are due to Alzheimer's rather than something else. For example, the risk of developing Alzheimer's disease between ages 65 and 70 without a family history is about 1.5%, whereas the risk for those with a family history rises to between 3% and 6%. But just because there is an increase in risk with a family history doesn't mean you will develop Alzheimer's if you have a family history of the disease. There are certainly many people with a family history of Alzheimer's who never develop the disease themselves.

We also know that some people have genetic differences that cause either too much beta amyloid to be formed or not enough to be cleared. The most common genetic variation that can lead to Alzheimer's disease is the APOE-e4 gene, which appears to be related to reduced clearance of beta amyloid. This gene is a major reason that individuals with a family history of Alzheimer's are more likely to develop the disease themselves. But we do not recommend testing for it, as it cannot determine whether Alzheimer's disease is present or not, nor whether it will develop in the future.

IN SPECIAL CIRCUMSTANCES A LUMBAR PUNCTURE CAN HELP TO CONFIRM ALZHEIMER'S DISEASE

Most cases of Alzheimer's disease can be correctly diagnosed with the standard evaluation described in *Chapter 1*. However, when Alzheimer's disease is strongly suspected but there is something unusual at play, such as the individual being younger than age 65 or there are early changes in movement or behavior, the doctor may recommend a lumbar puncture to analyze the levels of beta amyloid and tau in the spinal fluid. We don't use this test routinely both because it is not needed in the majority of individuals when the diagnosis is straight-forward, and because the test provides the right answer about 85 to 90% of the time but can be inconclusive 10 to 15% of the time.

A lumbar puncture—more commonly known as a spinal tap—may sound frightening, but it is actually a very safe and simple test that is less painful for most people than having an IV (intravenous line or catheter) placed. If the doctor suggests this test, your loved one would begin by either sitting or lying down on their side with their back to the doctor, and curling into a little ball by bringing their shoulders down and their knees up. The doctor would find the right spot, clean the area well, give them some numbing medicine (like in the dentist's office), insert a very thin needle, and take a small amount of spinal fluid out in order to test the levels of beta amyloid and tau.

AMYLOID AND TAU PET SCANS CAN CONFIRM ALZHEIMER'S DISEASE BUT ARE NOT PAID FOR BY MEDICARE OR OTHER INSURANCE

Amyloid and tau positron emission tomography or PET scans can correctly identify when the plaques and tangles of Alzheimer's disease are present 90% to 95% of the time. Most often, however, the diagnosis of Alzheimer's is clear and these scans are not needed. As with the lumbar puncture, when circumstances are unusual, these PET scans can be helpful to make sure that the diagnosis is correct. Both special tests provide similar information; choosing one versus the other is based on cost and availability.

A PET scan is like an "inside-out" X-ray. With an X-ray, the radiation beams go from the transmitter through the body and are collected on a film or X-ray detector. With amyloid and tau PET scans, the radiation is built into a tiny molecule that is engineered to stick to amyloid plaques or tau tangles. The molecule is injected through an IV in the arm, and if there are any amyloid plaques or tau tangles in the brain, it will stick to them. The radiation of the molecule sticking to the plaques is then detected on the X-ray detector.

Currently, amyloid and tau PET scans are not paid for by Medicare or other health insurance because they have not been proven to be cost-effective. If research studies (which are currently in progress) prove that PET scans are cost-effective, it is likely that they will be more widely used in the future. One way to obtain an amyloid or tau PET scan without cost is to participate in research; many clinical trials evaluating new treatments for Alzheimer's disease include a PET scan free of charge.

REDUCE YOUR RISK OF ALZHEIMER'S DISEASE BY DOING AEROBIC EXERCISE, EATING A HEALTHY DIET, AND BEING SOCIALLY ACTIVE

Want to reduce your own risk of developing Alzheimer's disease? There is increasing evidence that several lifestyle choices, including engaging in regular aerobic exercise, eating a Mediterranean-style diet, and staying socially and cognitively active, can help to keep your thinking and memory as strong as possible. You can learn more about these lifestyle choices in our book *Seven Steps to Managing Your Memory*.

SUMMARY

Alzheimer's is a disease in which amyloid plaques build up in the brain. The plaques damage brain cells, the cells develop tangles, and the tangles destroy the cells. Alzheimer's disease begins silently and progresses through very mild, mild, moderate, and severe stages. Age, being a woman, and family history are risk factors for the disease. Tests using a lumbar puncture or PET scan can help to confirm the diagnosis of Alzheimer's disease, but they are only used in special circumstances. Lastly, you can reduce your risk of developing Alzheimer's disease by eating a Mediterranean-style diet, engaging in aerobic exercise, and staying socially active.

Let's consider some examples to illustrate what we learned in this chapter.

- *Your friend told you that there is nothing you can do about Alzheimer's disease because if we live long enough everyone will get it. Is that true?*
  - No. Alzheimer's disease is more common in aging, but many people live to age 90 or 100 without the disease. Aerobic exercise, healthy eating, and social activities can all help reduce one's chances of developing Alzheimer's disease.

- *My loved one has dementia but there is no family history of Alzheimer's disease. Does that mean there must be some other cause of their dementia?*
  - Although the risk is less without a family history, everyone is at risk for Alzheimer's disease as they get older, so it still may be the cause of their dementia. You don't need a family history of Alzheimer's to get the disease.
- *My loved one has dementia and we can afford to get one of those PET scans. Should we just have the doctor order one and not bother with the rest of the evaluation?*
  - No. Even if the scan suggests Alzheimer's disease, there could still be many other treatable factors impairing their memory (such as a thyroid disorder, vitamin deficiency, or medication side effect) that can only be identified during the regular evaluation.
- *I'd really like to get one of those PET scans for my loved one, but I cannot afford it. What can I do?*
  - Participating in research is one way to obtain an amyloid or tau PET scan free of charge. The scan is included in many clinical trials evaluating new Alzheimer's medications.

3

Which other disorders cause dementia?

Having learned about Alzheimer's disease in *Chapter 2*, we're ready to discuss other common disorders that can cause dementia, including cerebrovascular disease (also known as strokes), dementia with Lewy bodies, frontotemporal dementia, primary progressive aphasia, and normal pressure hydrocephalus. Rarer causes of dementia, including alcohol-related dementia, chronic traumatic encephalopathy (CTE), corticobasal degeneration, human immunodeficiency virus (HIV) disease, multiple sclerosis, posterior cortical atrophy, progressive supranuclear palsy, and others, are described in the *Glossary* at the end of the book.

VASCULAR DEMENTIA IS DEMENTIA DUE TO STROKES

"Hi everyone, I'm Sara, and my father, Jack, has both Alzheimer's and vascular dementia. When he was diagnosed, we never thought he had a stroke, but the doctor said she could see lots of little strokes on the MRI. However, in the last couple of years he had three strokes that we brought him to the hospital for. The first caused slurred speech. The second made his face droop and he kept dropping things out of his right hand. The third was really weird—he didn't notice things on his left side, didn't even shave the left side of his face! Luckily, each of these strokes got better after a few days, although the problems can come out again if he gets sick or is really tired. But the thing I really want to talk about is that I can't help getting angry at him for doing stupid things, like leaving the stove on or getting lost. I know it's from the dementia, but I can't help feeling annoyed. And then I feel guilty about having those feelings," she finishes, her voice cracking.

Strokes, also called vascular disease or cerebrovascular disease because the problem is with blood vessels of the brain or "cerebrum," occur when an artery sending blood from the heart to the brain becomes blocked off, and part of the brain doesn't receive enough blood and dies.

Although individuals and family members usually notice major strokes from the blockage of large arteries right away, tiny strokes from the blockage of small and microscopic arteries in the brain are typically silent and go unnoticed until a brain imaging study such as an MRI or CT scan is performed and shows these small-vessel-disease strokes. Most people, in fact, have a handful of tiny strokes by the time they are in their 70s and 80s. These tiny strokes are generally too small to cause dementia all by themselves, but they can make thinking and memory worse when other disorders, such as Alzheimer's disease, are present. It is only when large numbers of these tiny strokes accumulate, or when the strokes are medium or large, that they cause vascular dementia.

If your loved one has any of the following major risk factors, they are at increased risk for strokes and vascular dementia:

Medical factors
- Prior stroke
- Prior stroke warning sign (transient ischemic attack or "TIA")
- Heart disease
- Disease of other blood vessels of the body
- Diabetes

- High cholesterol
- High blood pressure

Lifestyle factors
- Smoking
- Sedentary lifestyle
- Unhealthy diet
- Obesity
- Alcohol intake of more than one drink per day

Uncontrollable factors
- Old age: after age 55, the stroke risk doubles every decade

The good news is that, with the exception of age, you can help your loved one take charge of their life and reduce their risk of strokes. Work with their doctor to make sure that their medical conditions are under good control. If they are smoking, encourage them to quit today. Help them exercise for better health, eat a healthy diet, and keep a healthy weight. If they drink alcohol, make sure they drink in moderation—no more than one drink per day.

DEMENTIA WITH LEWY BODIES: FEATURES OF PARKINSON'S DISEASE, VISUAL HALLUCINATIONS, AND ACTING-OUT DREAMS

"My name is Martin, and Nina, my wife, also has two diseases. She has Alzheimer's and she also has dementia with Lewy bodies. When it started, Nina was having difficulty paying the bills and balancing the checkbook. She would also forget things—that's from the Alzheimer's. But then she began waking me up, saying, 'There's a dog in our bedroom!' I'd turn on the light and we'd look around together and there would never be a dog. She also began to move her arms and legs while she was sleeping like the dog was chasing her! You see, she was acting out her dreams. Then her walking became slow and shuffling, her writing shrank, and her hands started shaking. Now we're struggling with the basics, like dressing and getting to the bathroom on time. The main thing I'm worrying about is: How long can I keep this up? I'm barely getting any sleep, I'm doing laundry twice a day, and I'm no spring chicken myself."

Dementia with Lewy bodies is a common cause of dementia. It gets its name because of an abnormal collection of protein that interferes with brain cell function, seen only under the microscope. Lewy bodies are also present in Parkinson's disease, the difference being that in Parkinson's disease the Lewy bodies are only found in a part of the brain related to movement that causes tremor, slowness of movements, shuffling walking, reduced size of letters in writing, and diminished facial expression. In dementia with Lewy bodies, the Lewy bodies have spread throughout the brain and, in addition to the features of Parkinson's disease, they often cause trouble with vision—including visual hallucinations—and acting-out dreams at night. There may also be dramatic fluctuations in attention and alertness from one day to the next. Some people who have been living with Parkinson's disease for many years will later develop dementia with Lewy bodies. Because it started with Parkinson's disease, in these individuals it is sometimes called Parkinson's disease dementia instead of dementia with Lewy bodies.

In pure dementia with Lewy bodies, the primary cognitive difficulty is with vision, attention, and performing complicated activities. Although there can be difficulty forming and retrieving memories, once memories are formed they should not be lost. However, it is very common to have both dementia with Lewy bodies and Alzheimer's disease. These individuals have the features of both diseases.

Common features of dementia with Lewy bodies are as follows:

Features of Parkinson's disease
- Tremor
- Slow, shuffling walking
- Falls
- Slowness of movement
- Difficulty rising from a low chair, car seat, or toilet
- Reduced size of letters in writing
- Diminished facial expression

Visual disturbances
- Visual hallucinations of people or animals
- Difficulty seeing

Acting-out dreams

Fluctuations in attention and alertness
- There may be dramatic variation in abilities between one day and another.

Thinking and memory problems
- Poor attention
- Difficulty with complicated activities
- Difficulty forming and retrieving memories

FRONTOTEMPORAL DEMENTIA AFFECTS PERSONALITY, BEHAVIOR, AND COGNITION

After Martin finishes, a middle-aged woman in the group starts speaking.

"My husband was diagnosed with frontotemporal dementia at age 55, and it began with him becoming a jerk. For example, not only did he no longer hold open the door for me, he would go through first and let it slam in my face. If he didn't like what I was watching on TV, he would just change the channel without asking me. He purchased a fancy new car that we couldn't afford. Then he began to eat things—like a tub of ice cream or a whole box of cookies—in bed while I was trying to sleep. But the thing that really upset me is that around that time I was diagnosed with cancer and he really didn't care. He just complained that my chemotherapy schedule was interfering with him getting to his golf game. All this took me by surprise, because my husband always used to be so sweet. But it came on so slowly that I just thought, 'Here's that midlife crisis men go through.' And this is all happening in his 50s—it never occurred to me that it was some kind of dementia. I finally figured out something was wrong with him when he stopped playing golf—and then he stopped going to work. All he wanted to do was sit on the couch, stare at the TV, and eat—anything: a box of cake mix, a tin of frosting, or a jar of mayonnaise. And he didn't even care if the TV was on or not—he would stare at it either way. That's when I took him to his doctor. I feel so guilty for thinking he was just being a jerk and not bringing him to the doctor sooner! The biggest problem I'm dealing with now is that when he wants to urinate he will just do it wherever he is. He won't bother going into the bathroom or pulling down his pants. And when I tell him we need to go change him into clean clothes, he argues with me!"

Frontotemporal dementia usually looks different than Alzheimer's disease and other causes of dementia in a few ways. Most people with frontotemporal dementia start to show symptoms between the ages of 45 and 65, although in about one-quarter of individuals the disease is first detected after age 65. Additionally, the most prominent symptoms are personality and behavior changes and trouble performing complicated activities. Friends and family members of individuals with frontotemporal dementia frequently describe them as behaving like "different people." They often show socially inappropriate behaviors (such as making sexually explicit comments), have poor manners, make impulsive decisions, and engage in careless actions. They frequently show little sympathy or empathy for others. Loss of interest, drive, and motivation to do anything is very common. Some individuals compulsively perform repetitive movements, such as turning the light switch off and on whenever they walk by it. Others show a marked change in food preferences (often preferring sweets) or engage in binge eating, excessive smoking, or drinking alcohol. Individuals with frontotemporal dementia are unable to realize or understand that anything is wrong with their behavior; it is family or friends who bring the abnormal behavior to medical attention. Changes in memory are related to difficulty paying attention, which impairs the formation of new memories and the ability to retrieve them. Performing complicated activities becomes difficult, such as using a new software program, preparing a gourmet meal, balancing the checkbook, and setting up an electronic gadget.

Common features of frontotemporal dementia are as follows:

General features
- Three-quarters of individuals present between the ages of 45 to 65.
- Prominent change in personality—individual often seems like a different person

Changes in behavior
- Socially inappropriate behavior, including insensitive social remarks
- Loss of manners
- Impulsive, rash, or careless actions

Apathy or inertia
- Loss of interest, drive, or motivation
- Decreased initiation of activity
- Neglect of self-care

Loss of sympathy or empathy
- Diminished response to other people's needs or feelings
- Diminished social interest, interrelatedness, personal warmth, and social engagement

Perseverative, stereotyped, or compulsive/ritualistic behavior
- Simple repetitive movements
- Compulsive or ritualistic behaviors
- Repeating the same words

Abnormal eating behavior
- Altered food preferences
- Binge eating or increased use of alcohol or cigarettes
- Putting inedible objects in mouth

Thinking and memory problems
- Poor attention
- Difficulty with complicated activities
- Difficulty forming and retrieving memories

PRIMARY PROGRESSIVE APHASIA AFFECTS SPEECH AND LANGUAGE

"With my wife," the next member in the group begins, "the problem is with words. It began when she couldn't find the words she was looking for. So, my kids and I began to jump in and finish her sentences for her. We didn't think much of it—I mean, I've got trouble coming up with names myself. But then she started not knowing what the words mean. We were talking with our granddaughter about going to the zoo, and she says she's excited to see the giraffes. My wife looks at me and asks, 'What's a giraffe?' Then in October we're getting ready to go buy a pumpkin and she says, 'Pumpkin? What's a pumpkin?' I mean, she's lived in New England all her life—grew up with Halloween. That's when I started to get scared. We knew something was wrong. Now she really doesn't have any language left. But the funny thing is, somehow we can still communicate. With her face and gestures and the movements she makes, I'm able to figure out what she wants—most of the time, anyways—and she always knows when to give me a hug."

Difficulty finding the names of people, places, and other proper nouns is frequently seen in normal aging. When there is trouble finding ordinary words or difficulty with other parts of speech and language, however, it could be a sign of dementia. Although speech and language problems are most often seen in common disorders of thinking and memory such as Alzheimer's disease and vascular dementia, there are some individuals who present first and foremost with speech and language problems. These individuals have primary progressive aphasia.

Primary progressive aphasia has three common variants. In the logopenic (word-finding) variant, the difficulty is mainly finding and pronouncing words, with comprehension and grammar being normal. In the semantic (word-meaning) variant, there is difficulty naming objects, comprehending single words, and even understanding what objects are used for. In the non-fluent/agrammatic variant, there is effortful, halting speech with errors, distortions, and impaired grammar; comprehension is normal for simple sentences but may be impaired for complicated ones.

Common features of primary progressive aphasia are as follows:

General features
- Difficulty with language is the most prominent feature, particularly at the start
- Language problems impair daily living activities

Logopenic (word-finding) variant
- Difficulty retrieving single words in ordinary speech and when naming items
- Pronunciation errors are common
- Difficulty repeating phrases and sentences is common
- Comprehension is normal
- Use of grammar is normal

Semantic (word-meaning) variant
- Naming objects is impaired
- Comprehension is impaired, even of single words
- Comprehension is often impaired for what some objects are, not just their names
- Difficulty reading and writing is common

Non-fluent/agrammatic variant
- Speech takes great effort and is halting, with speech errors and distortions
- Grammar is impaired
- Comprehension of complex sentences may be impaired

NORMAL PRESSURE HYDROCEPHALUS IS CHARACTERIZED BY DIFFICULTY WALKING, URINARY URGENCY OR INCONTINENCE, AND POOR ATTENTION

Normal pressure hydrocephalus (often referred to by its initials, NPH) generally starts with a slowing of the walking; small steps; slow, multi-step turns; poor balance; and a need to run to the bathroom to urinate. It is caused by an excess of fluid in the brain. Studies show that after treatment with a shunt (a tube that drains the excess fluid), the deterioration of thinking and memory is halted and there is improvement in the walking and the urgent need to urinate.

Common thinking and memory problems that occur in normal pressure hydrocephalus include poor attention, being easily distracted, difficulty performing complicated tasks, loss of interest in activities, and slowness in thought and movement. It is difficult to pay attention when new memories are being formed and retrieved.

Normal pressure hydrocephalus is an uncommon disorder and, in the end, all dementias lead to problems with thinking and memory, walking, and urinary incontinence. But because normal pressure hydrocephalus can often be successfully treated, stopping the decline in function, it is always worth considering.

SUMMARY

In addition to Alzheimer's disease, other brain disorders of aging that affect thinking and memory include vascular dementia, dementia with Lewy bodies, frontotemporal dementia, primary progressive aphasia, and normal pressure hydrocephalus. Each produces characteristic changes in thinking, memory, language, behavior, and/or movement that allow you and the doctor to know when to consider them as possible causes of your loved one's dementia.

Let's consider some examples to illustrate what we learned in this chapter.

- *You've seen your loved one's MRI report and it says they have "scattered T2 hyperintensities consistent with microvascular ischemic disease." What does that mean?*
  - That's a doctor's way of saying that there is something on the MRI scan that looks like tiny, small-vessel strokes.
- *Your loved one has never had a stroke, yet the doctor says they did and she can see it on the MRI scan. How can that be?*
  - Many strokes—especially small ones—are "silent," meaning that they may not cause any noticeable symptoms.
- *Your loved one has had several episodes of seeing a person or animal that isn't there when they were waking up or falling asleep. Does that mean they're going crazy?*
  - Not at all. Seeing people or animals that are not there may be a sign of dementia with Lewy bodies. Let the doctor know about these symptoms; there are medications that can help.
- *Your loved one has trouble finding words. Does that mean they have primary progressive aphasia?*
  - Not necessarily. Although it is possible they have primary progressive aphasia, because word-finding difficulties occur so frequently, it could be part of a more common disorder such Alzheimer's disease or vascular dementia.
- *Your loved one's walking has become very slow and they need to rush to urinate. Should you speak with the doctor about whether they might have normal pressure hydrocephalus?*
  - Yes. Normal pressure hydrocephalus is one of the most treatable causes of dementia. The outcomes are better when it is detected and treated early, so make an appointment for them to see the doctor today.
- *You've noticed that your wife, age 57, is acting odd. Previously a considerate person, she now says what she thinks without concern of whether it would hurt someone's feelings. Although she used to be*

health conscious, she now wants to eat dessert for breakfast, lunch, and dinner. Lately, she has been stealing food off other people's plates at restaurants. What's going on?

○ If your loved one behaves in the way just described, make sure they see their doctor. Frontotemporal dementia, strokes, or a brain tumor are just some of the possible causes.

Step 2

MANAGE PROBLEMS

In *Step 1* we learned what dementia and Alzheimer's disease are and then reviewed other causes of dementia. In *Step 2* we will explore why memory, language, vision, emotions, behavior, sleep, and bodily functions become impaired in dementia, how these impairments lead to problems, and—most importantly—how to manage these problems. Before we dive in, we'd like to make two points: When dementia has reached the moderate or severe stage, the cognitive and other problems are generally similar regardless of its cause. However, every person with dementia is also different, and different people with dementia will experience different problems.

IN THEIR MODERATE TO SEVERE STAGES, MOST DEMENTIAS LOOK ALIKE

Because each cause of dementia tends to affect a different part of the brain first, each begins with a distinct profile of cognitive impairment and other problems. For example, Alzheimer's disease starts with memory problems, primary progressive aphasia starts with language problems, and frontotemporal dementia starts with behavior problems. However, as these disorders and other dementias progress, more and more brain regions become affected, so that by the time these dementias have reached the moderate or severe stage, they often look similar to each other, and memory, language, vision, emotions, behavior, sleep, and bodily functions are all impaired. It is for this reason that when we are discussing the problems that occur in dementia and their solutions, we can discuss them in general—regardless of which disease is causing the dementia.

EVERY INDIVIDUAL WITH DEMENTIA IS DIFFERENT

Having stated clearly that individuals with moderate to severe dementia may experience similar problems regardless of which disease they have, we also want to state clearly that every person is different—each with their own abilities, talents, fears, and limitations—and how the dementia affects each person may also be different. For these reasons it is not possible to predict precisely which problems any one individual will experience.

In *Step 2* we describe a large number of problems that commonly occur in dementia. Rest assured that we do not expect that your loved one will have all or even half of these problems. We tried to be exhaustive, however, so that if they do exhibit a problem, you will be armed with the knowledge you need to understand and manage that problem.

4

How to approach problems in dementia

Although many specific problems in dementia are best managed by equally specific solutions, there are some general approaches that can be used in a wide range of situations. In this chapter we will review three general approaches:

1. We will discuss how to better understand behaviors by examining what happened before the behavior and what came after it.
2. We will review four easy-to-remember tips that you can use in the heat of the moment when things are not going well.
3. We will consider three timely suggestions to improve communication with your loved one.

THE *ABCs OF BEHAVIOR CHANGE*: ANTECEDENTS, BEHAVIORS, CONSEQUENCES

All behaviors have a purpose. Do you find this statement surprising? The purpose of a behavior may be to express an emotion, such as frustration or anger. It may be to satisfy a need, such as hunger or affection. It could even be to communicate information, such as "I want to be left alone" or "I want to stay in the car."

In order to manage problem behaviors, you first need to understand the purpose behind them. The *ABCs of Behavior Change* provides a framework for understanding why problem behaviors occur. You can identify the *antecedent*: what was happening with your loved one or in the environment *before* a behavior occurred. You can also identify the *consequence*: what happened *after* the behavior occurred. Keeping a log that identifies the antecedents and consequences surrounding problem behavior will enable you to identify patterns that tell you why the behavior is occurring, select an intervention to try to improve the behavior, apply that intervention, and reassess to determine if the intervention is working or whether you need to try something different.

Behaviors are observable and can be measured

A *behavior* is something that is specific and observable. It is something that your loved one does or does not do. Behaviors can be seen, heard, or felt. Behaviors are not things we assume or infer. For example, when we see our loved one yelling, we might assume they are angry, but anger is not a behavior. Anger is an emotion we assume our loved one is feeling when we see they are yelling. The specific behavior that we observe is yelling. Said another way, yelling is a behavior because it is specific and observable—something we can hear and see.

Because behaviors are specific and observable, we can measure them: how often they occur (their frequency) and/ or how long they occur for (their duration). We may want to decrease certain behaviors (such as yelling or asking repetitive questions) and increase other behaviors (such as sleeping or bathing).

Antecedents come before behaviors

Antecedents are the things happening with your loved one or in the environment *before* a behavior occurs. Antecedents can include events (bath time or bed time), circumstances (noises or crowds), or objects (car keys or photographs). Antecedents can also be less apparent, including things like time of day, season, or physical discomfort. When trying to identify antecedents, in addition to the more obvious environmental triggers, it can be helpful to consider two other categories: physical and emotional needs. Your loved one may have trouble communicating their needs and may act out to get them met. Physical needs can include hunger and thirst, pain and discomfort, and over- or under-stimulation. Perhaps they are constipated or feeling ill. Maybe they are itchy from tags on clothing. Or the environment may be too noisy—or too quiet. Emotional needs can include a desire for affection, company, space, new people or places, or a change in routine. When we are trying to identify antecedents, we might ask ourselves these questions:

- What day and time of day was it?
- What was the environment like?
- Who was there?
- Was there something happening or about to happen?
- Was there something your loved one wanted, like food or drink?

These questions can help us to identify aspects of the environment or unmet physical or emotional needs that might be causing the problem behavior. These questions may help you discover, for example, that the yelling always occurs at bath time.

Consequences occur after behaviors

Consequences are things that occur immediately after the behavior. They can be something you do or something that happens in the environment. Remember, all behaviors have a purpose. Identifying the consequence of the behavior may help you understand its purpose. When we are trying to identify consequences, we might ask ourselves these questions:

- How did the environment change?
- Did something start or stop as a result of the behavior?
- Did your loved one get something like food, drink, or attention?

For example, was the consequence of the yelling that you decided to skip the bath that day? Note that not every consequence or antecedent needs to provide an explanation for a behavior. Part of identifying them is to enable you to figure out which are relevant and which are not.

Creating a behavior log

Behavior logs can help you to identify the antecedents and consequences of behaviors and, importantly, help you to track them to see if your interventions are successfully reducing unwanted behaviors and increasing desired ones. Behavior logs can also show you that sometimes our actions can accidentally make things worse!

Why would a behavior get worse? Well, if your loved one yells every time you try to give them a bath until you give up and skip the bath, they may "learn" that they can avoid things they don't like by yelling. They may then start yelling when you ask them to do other things they don't want to do, such as get dressed or get out of the car.

Using the example above, let's complete a behavior log.

Antecedents	Behavior	Consequence
(Include the date, time of day, place, person[s] present, and events)	(specific, observable, measurable—frequency and/or duration)	(How did things change?)
Sunday, 3 PM *Me & my loved one* *Bath time*	*Yelling for 7 minutes*	*Decided to skip the bath that day*

Use the *ABCs of Behavior Change* to change behaviors

Once you are able to identify antecedents, behaviors, and consequences, you can begin to try to change the behavior. For example, you want your loved one to decrease (or stop) yelling. Then you need to decide what you want your loved one to do instead, the desired behavior—in this case, take a bath. The next step involves some creativity. To choose an intervention, you need to decide how you are going to change the environment to result in the desired behavior. There may be many things you can try to change, but it is important to only make one change at a time so that you know what worked and what didn't. In order to help your loved one take a bath without yelling, instead of asking them to get ready to take a bath, you might instead make small requests, like asking them to sit on a stool by the tub and put their feet in the warm water. If this intervention works, they are no longer yelling, and now they're happy to slip into the tub and wash up, that's great; you can stop there! If it doesn't, you need to reassess the intervention and try something new. For example, maybe next time you'll try playing their favorite music in the bathroom.

Practice makes perfect; enlist family and friends to help

Martin sighs as Nina begins to noisily tap the coffee table. He looks at the clock: 2:00 PM. He tries to recall what time Nina fell back asleep: *Maybe 4 AM?* Then she slept until 10 AM, missing breakfast.

Soon Nina is slapping the coffee table. Sighing again, Martin gets up and says to Nina, "Would you like something to eat?" She immediately stands up and they go into the kitchen, where he makes her a sandwich. She devours it hungrily.

Despite sleeping late, Nina seems tired at her usual 3 PM nap time. Martin lays down with her and within minutes she is asleep.

Martin thinks about everything that just happened and writes it out in a behavior log:

Antecedents	Behavior	Consequence
Trouble sleeping at night, slept late, skipped breakfast, and had an early lunch	*At 2 PM began noisily tapping and then slapping the coffee table for 15 minutes until I offered her a snack*	*Made her a sandwich and then laid down with her on the bed and she took a nap*

> Looking at the behavior log, Martin ponders how he might be able to reduce Nina's tapping and slapping in the future. Then he slaps his own forehead as he suddenly realizes that Nina's tapping may be her way of letting him know that she is tired and hungry! He sees how she didn't sleep well the night before and skipped breakfast. And she stopped tapping after she ate and took a nap. Now he knows what to do next time: Help Nina get a good night's sleep and make sure she gets a snack if she misses a meal.

Using the *ABCs of Behavior Change* takes practice. You should start by keeping a log of your own that includes the antecedents, behaviors, and consequences, like the one that Martin did. Then you can pick an intervention and try to find something that works. Don't get discouraged—the first intervention you try might not work. You also don't need to try to figure out an intervention alone. This is a great time to involve your care team: family, friends, and professionals who can help you think of interventions you can try. See *Step 4* for learning more about how to create your care team.

THE *4Rs*: REASSURE, RECONSIDER, REDIRECT, AND RELAX

Using the *ABCs of Behavior Change* method is an ideal way to understand and improve behaviors when you have some time to step back and consider each behavior thoughtfully. When you are in the midst of dealing with a situation, however, it is not necessarily the best time to start filling in a behavior log.

At that time, we suggest the *4Rs*: reassure, reconsider, redirect, and relax. We want to *reassure* our loved one that everything is alright. We want to *reconsider* the situation from their point of view. We want to *redirect* them to activities that they enjoy and are calming. And we want to remember that it is important that we *relax* so that we do not inadvertently escalate the situation.

Reassure

Martin looks at the clock as he is slicing vegetables: *5 o'clock.* He knows this is the time that Nina will often wander out of the house. Just as he is thinking these thoughts, he hears the front door open. He sets down the knife and rushes to the front door.

Standing in her slippers, Nina is staring outside. She looks at Martin as he approaches but doesn't seem to recognize him. She starts to shuffle out of the house.

"There, there, girl, everything's OK," Martin says as he reaches out and starts rubbing her back. "You're home, Nina." After another minute of rubbing her back and using reassuring words, she follows him back into the house.

Martin considers the *4Rs* and realizes that he has been reassuring Nina all along without even thinking about it.

It is important to understand that your loved one with dementia may have difficulty interacting with the world around them. Because of their memory loss, people and things once familiar may become unfamiliar. Noise, crowds, and activity may be difficult to understand, and they may feel easily overwhelmed. They may be worried or scared when they can't see you—thinking you've been gone for hours even if it's only been a few minutes. In short, there are many reasons why an individual with dementia may feel anxious and afraid, even if they have never had trouble with these emotions before. It can be helpful to remind yourself that if your loved one is yelling or acting agitated, it may be related to their feeling afraid or nervous. Reassure them that everything is alright. Phrases like, "You're safe," "Everything is OK," and "I'm here for you" can provide comfort. You may need to reassure them repeatedly. Reassurance from you can help reduce or stop many problem behaviors.

Reconsider

"Dad!" Sara shouts as she knocks on his front door. "Please come out to dinner with us. We would love to see you. It's not good for you to stay in the house by yourself all the time."

"I don't want to go out," Jack says through the door. "Remember what happened last time."

Sara rolls her eyes, thinking about how astounding it is that her father has such a hard time remembering most things, yet he still remembers that awful lunch as if it happened yesterday: He had trouble understanding the waiter, reading the menu, remembering what he wanted to order, and pronouncing the name of the entrée.

She lifts up her hand to bang on the door again and insist that Jack come out, when she remembers the 4Rs. *Reconsider,* she thinks. *I need to consider how my father feels in this situation. Although it won't bother me if he has trouble ordering in a restaurant, he might feel frustrated and embarrassed.*

It is important to consider your loved one's perspective. Their experience of situations might be very different than you might imagine. For example, perhaps your loved one becomes angry every time the home health aide visits and tries to help him bathe. This behavior may seem mysterious, but reconsidering things from his perspective may help explain it. Because of his memory loss, he may perceive the aide as a complete stranger—even though she has been bathing him for months! He also may not remember that he needs help bathing. So, from his perspective, a stranger is asking him to take his clothes off so she can bathe him, and he may feel outraged, anxious, or confused. Reconsidering the situation from your loved one's point of view can improve your ability to empathize with them, help you feel calmer, and provide you with clues about what you might be able to do to manage the problem behavior.

Redirect

On another day, Nina is again wandering out of the house.

"Come on, Nina, everything is OK," Martin says reassuringly as he rubs her back and gently tries to pull her back into the house. "Let's go back inside."

Nina starts to shuffle down the steps away from him.

Martin thinks through the 4Rs. *Reassure: I'm doing that. Reconsider: From her point of view, she doesn't realize she's already home, although I've tried to explain that she is. OK, the next R is . . . redirect: I need to direct her attention to something that will get her inside.*

"Hey, girl, you know what we have inside the house? We've got lots of fun things! If you're hungry, I've got some delicious fruit that you can snack on, or we can have a little cheese and crackers, whatever you like."

Nina turns to look at Martin, clearly interested in what he's saying.

"And if you'd like to listen to some music or do a little dancing, we've got all our old records—come with me and let's pick out one to put on the stereo."

Together they walk back inside the house.

Simply telling your loved one to stop a problem behavior rarely works. Redirecting them to something they like often does. When you redirect your loved one, you change the focus and direct them from the upsetting or counterproductive event or environment to something else. This change may be accomplished by taking your loved one into a different room, starting a fun conversation or activity, pointing out something interesting, or giving your loved one a novel, interesting, comforting, or well-loved object. Use a nurturing touch and tone of voice to redirect your loved one. Using a loud or harsh tone will generally escalate the behavior, which brings us to our last R—relax.

Relax

Sara reflects upon what she learned by reconsidering how her father must feel when he has difficulty ordering in a restaurant. She realizes that she is upset—upset at her father for never wanting to leave his house, upset at herself for not being able to get him out, and also upset at herself because she never really thought about how he must be feeling. She knows she needs to use the fourth R, relax.

Sara takes in a deep breath, trying to relax. Nothing happens; she still feels annoyed.

She tries counting to 10. This helps her feel a little bit calmer.

Sara knocks on Jack's door. After a minute, he opens it slowly and looks at her.

"Dad," she says calmly, "what about if we got some takeout and brought it over. Would that be OK?"

"Thanks, that would be fine," he says. "I just don't want to be in a restaurant and have to make those decisions and talk to the waiter and stuff."

With diminishing abilities, your loved one may increasingly rely on you to help them interpret the world around them. Consciously or unconsciously, they may use your emotions as a way to know how they should be feeling and responding. If you are anxious and upset—whether because of their behavior or something else—your loved one may feed off of your feelings and also become anxious and upset. Even if the words you are using are reassuring, if your tone of voice or body language reflects that you're feeling frustrated or angry, your loved is likely to pick up on these nonverbal signals. This is why it is so important that you remain calm and relaxed—especially when faced with problem behavior.

Of course, it isn't always easy to relax your posture, uncross your arms, loosen your hands, and speak calmly and reassuringly. Remaining relaxed in the face of aggressive, agitated, embarrassing, and irritating behaviors is hard for everyone. Practicing good self-care will make it easier for you to remain calm and collected when your loved one is not. Learning deep-breathing and relaxation techniques can help you control your emotions. In *Step 4* we will discuss these and other ways that you can take care of yourself, which will help you to be able to remain calm even in the most challenging situations.

IMPROVE COMMUNICATION WITH YOUR LOVED ONE: THE *THREE TIME PRINCIPLES*

The final broad strategy for managing problems is to communicate with your loved one as effectively as possible. Because they may be experiencing changes in their memory, attention, language, and vision, communication is more difficult. This difficulty alone will often cause frustration and create behavior problems. Practicing good communication skills can foster positive behaviors and reduce challenging ones. We suggest the *Three Time Principles*:

1. Take your time
2. One thing at a time
3. Offer timely praise

Take your time

"I'm sorry that I have to run, Dad," Sara says as she puts on her coat. "Don't forget that I'm picking you up on Tuesday for your hearing appointment at 10 o'clock," she says over her shoulder

as she walks to the front door, "and you've got your appointment with the eye doctor at noon on Thursday," she says, opening the door. "Oh, and let me know if you need anything from
the store," she finishes as she starts to shut the door.

"Umm . . ." Jack begins. "Can you say that one more time? When
are you picking me up for what?"

"Sorry, Dad, got to run," she says, shutting the door.

As she is driving home, she worries that Jack won't remember everything she just told him. *Hmm*, she thinks. *Maybe I should have taken
my time, not rushed, and made sure Dad was paying attention.*

When communicating with your loved one, allow sufficient
time for unhurried interactions. It is always helpful to begin by
making eye contact to ensure they are paying attention. Gentle
physical touch, like a hand on their shoulder, may help to focus
their attention. Reducing any distractions in the environment
can also be useful. It is important to always use a soothing
voice, a pleasant expression, and comforting body language.

One thing at a time

"Do you want to help with breakfast?" Martin asks.

Nina nods her head.

"Alright! While I'm cutting the fruit, why don't you put the bread in
the toaster and put the jam and butter on the table?"

As Martin resumes cutting the fruit, Nina shuffles toward the
breadbox, stops, shuffles toward the refrigerator, stops, turns,
and looks at Martin.

"What's the matter?" he says, seeing Nina standing in the middle
of the floor. *Oh, one thing at a time*, he remembers. "Please put
the bread in the toaster," he says clearly while motioning with
his hand toward the breadbox and the toaster next to it.

He watches as Nina shuffles over and, one slice at a time, puts
the bread into the toaster and then pushes the lever down. She
turns to him.

"Now you can go over to the refrigerator," he says.

As your loved one's dementia progresses, you may find it helpful to slow down your speech and speak deliberately and clearly. Because their understanding of language may be impaired, use your tone of voice, facial expression, as well as hand and arm gestures to help them to know what you are trying to say. As it becomes more difficult for them to follow complicated, multistep commands, it will be important to break tasks down into simple, one-step commands when asking them to do something.

For example, instead of asking your loved one to get undressed, get into the shower, and wash their hair, it may be better to say each of these steps separately, adding the next request only after the prior one has been successfully completed. Begin with "get undressed" or maybe just "take off your shirt," and, after that step has been completed, proceed with the next step. Similarly, favorite hobbies that require multiple steps (such as cooking or gardening) are often given up as the dementia takes hold but may possibly be resumed (with a bit of supervision) if they are broken down into individual steps.

Offer timely praise

In general, avoid criticizing your loved one's behavior and provide praise generously. Offering praise and appreciation can protect against problem behavior. Find something genuine to praise, as exaggerated praise might seem insulting. There is almost always something to praise, even if it is just their effort in trying an activity. Remember, your loved one may feel insecure and uncertain, and giving sincere praise can help them feel valued and included. Fostering positive feelings helps prevent negative ones that can underlie behavior problems.

SUMMARY

There are several general strategies for managing problems in individuals with dementia. The *ABCs of Behavior Change* method identifies the antecedents and consequences surrounding a behavior, which can help you discover its cause, track it, and try different interventions to change it. The *4Rs*— reassure, reconsider, redirect, and relax—provide some rules of thumb that you can use even in the middle of a difficult situation. Lastly, the *Three Time Principles* can help you improve communication by taking your time, asking for only one thing at a time, and offering timely praise.

Let's consider some examples to illustrate what we learned in this chapter.

- *About an hour after the grandchildren come to visit, my wife becomes agitated. She used to love playing with them, but now she ends up yelling and saying nasty things. It upsets everyone and the visit often ends abruptly. I'm not sure what's wrong or what to do.*
  - Keeping a behavior log to identify the antecedents and consequences around the behavior can help you understand why your wife is becoming upset. Perhaps the grandchildren are visiting right before dinner so it is being served later than usual. Changing the time of the visit may reduce or eliminate the problem. There could be many other reasons, and a behavior log can provide clues for what to try next if the first intervention doesn't work.
- *My father doesn't want to get out of the car when we arrive at the doctor's office. I've tried pleading with him, talking sternly to him, and even trying to pull him out of the car. Once he started crying, and last time he tried to hit me. What should I do?*
  - Your father may be anxious about visiting the doctor, which may lead him to resist getting out of the car. When he sees you becoming frustrated, angry, and upset, it only makes him more agitated. Remember the *4Rs*: reassure, reconsider, redirect, and relax. Reassure him with soothing words. Reconsider things from his point of view: Your father doesn't understand why he needs to see the doctor if he doesn't feel sick. Redirect him to a pleasing activity such as getting out of the car for a walk, telling him a favorite story or joke, or playing some music he likes on

your phone. Stay relaxed and calm; it will help him become calm as well.

- *I asked my husband to wash his hands, set the table, fill the glasses with water, and then come help me in the kitchen. When I checked on him 20 minutes later he was watching TV. I could tell he washed his hands, but nothing else was done. So, I asked him again to set the table, fill the glasses, and then come help me. Fifteen minutes later the table was half-set, the water wasn't in the glasses, and he's agitated and storming around the dining room, periodically stopping to pound on the table. What should I do?*
  - As his dementia progresses, it can be difficult for your husband to follow multi-step commands. He may only remember one of the several things you asked him to do. This failure may cause him to feel embarrassed, frustrated, or annoyed, which can result in behavior problems such as anger and agitation. It is important to break larger tasks into small, one-step commands. You might ask your husband first to wash his hands, then set the table, then to fill the glasses, and finally to help you in the kitchen. Give him help with each step if he needs it Remember that steps like "set the table" can be broken down into smaller steps. Clear, one-step commands can reduce frustration and problem behavior.

5

How to manage memory problems

When memory fails it can cause many problems. Some problems, such as shadowing or repeating questions and stories, are fairly benign. Other problems, such as misplacing items or being disoriented for a few minutes, are usually not serious. But some problems, such as not taking medications properly or leaving the stove on, can have catastrophic consequences. In this chapter we will discuss why memory fails in dementia and methods to manage the more serious memory problems. Some of these methods are based on using brain systems that are relatively preserved in dementia to help those memory systems that are damaged, and other methods rely on you or a memory aid to compensate for the impaired memory of your loved one. Which methods you should try depends on how impaired their memory is, why their memory is impaired, as well as which memory issues are most problematic.

OLDER MEMORIES MAY BE PRESERVED IN DEMENTIA

Before we begin managing memory problems, we need to understand which memories tend to be impaired and which do not. For example, how is it that an individual with dementia who does not know where they are or what they had for breakfast that morning may still be able to remember their friends from high school? The answer is that memory for one's current location and breakfast is stored in the hippocampus, the brain's memory center, whereas older memories (such as those from high school) are stored in another region of the brain called the cortex. Although the hippocampus may be damaged early on, most causes of dementia do not affect the memory regions in the cortex until quite late in the disease.

This discrepancy between remembering things that happened long ago versus activities from the day or week before is often confusing. We've had many families tell us that, whatever is wrong with their loved one, they're sure it can't be Alzheimer's because they can still remember everything that happened 50 years ago. You now understand why remembering things that happened long ago may be preserved in Alzheimer's and other causes of dementia—at least for a while—because these older memories are stored in different parts of the brain. The memory problems in dementia are typically characterized by rapid forgetting of new information.

IMPAIRED ATTENTION MAY LEAD TO TROUBLE LEARNING AND RETRIEVING INFORMATION

Jack is taking a refresher pottery course at his local community center.

"Step 1," the teacher says, "is to pick your clay. Low-fire clays are great for . . ."

Buzz, buzz. Jack is distracted by a vibrating sound. *Buzz, buzz,* he hears again. *It sounds like a cellphone,* he thinks. He looks behind him, trying to determine where the sound is coming from.

"Step 2 is to determine which method you are going to use . . ."

Buzz, buzz. There it goes again! Jack thinks. Every minute or so he
    hears another buzz.
Well, that class was a waste of time, Jack thinks to himself as he gets
    into his car. *I couldn't pay attention with that cellphone buzzing all
    evening!* He begins driving toward home. *Buzz, buzz,* he hears—
    and feels! He pulls over to the side of the road and reaches
    into his coat pocket. There is his new cellphone, which he had
    forgotten all about. It buzzes again, and now he sees the text
    message his daughter Sara sent him: "Don't forget to go to your
    pottery class!"

Not paying enough attention is a common reason why people with dementia—and healthy individuals—have difficulty
remembering new information. For example, if you are watching the football game and another person comes into the room
and starts talking to you, you may not remember what the person said because you focused too much of your attention on
the game and too little on what the person was saying. Anyone
who is distracted and not paying attention will find it difficult
to remember new information.

Poor attention may also impair one's ability to retrieve
information. A common and normal occurrence is when you
walk into a room to do something but then cannot remember
what it was. What typically happens is that you walk in to get
a particular item, see something else that triggers a new and
different thought, become distracted, lose the focus of your
attention, and then cannot remember what you walked in to
get. For example, let's say that you are going to the basement to
change the laundry. You walk down the stairs and notice a box
with your favorite Tony Bennett record in it. Seeing the record
may distract you sufficiently such that you no longer remember
what you went downstairs to do. This disruption of attention
has interfered with your retrieval of the memory.

It turns out that attention is almost always impaired in dementia, causing people with dementia to frequently become distracted, stop paying attention, and experience difficulty learning and retrieving relevant information. Memory strategies and aids may be able to compensate for impaired attention.

IN MILD DEMENTIA, MEMORY STRATEGIES AND AIDS CAN HELP

Memory strategies (mental techniques) and aids (physical tools) may be able to help your loved one if their dementia is only in the mild stage (meaning that although they may have trouble preparing meals or managing money, they are still able to dress, bathe, eat neatly, and control their bowels and bladder).

Memory strategies can benefit those with mild memory problems

When memory problems are mild, the following strategies can help. (For more details on memory strategies and aids, please see our book *Seven Steps to Managing Your Memory*.)

  Practice active attention: Encourage your loved one to use conscious effort to pay attention to relevant details that need to be remembered, such as facts, names, or landmarks. Mindfulness training (through a class, book, or phone app) can improve one's ability to practice active attention.

  Minimize distractions in the environment: It is easier to focus on what one is trying to remember if there are fewer distractions. Turn off the telephone, television, radio, and email program.

  Take breaks: One can only pay full attention for so long before fatigue sets in. When it does, have them take a break.

  Repeat information spaced out over time: One of the most successful ways to remember information is to repeat it several times in a row, then again after a few minutes, again after an hour, again after a few more hours, and again before one goes to bed.

Continuing this repetition periodically over the next day, week, and month can help one remember information for a long time.

Make connections: Our brains are wired to form connections between information. Link something new that one is trying to remember to something that one already know well.

Create visual images: We all remember pictures better than words, so making mental images will help one remember things.

Put it in a location: To help remember a list of items, mentally place an item in each room (or each part of each room) in one's house. To retrieve the items, one simply walks through the house, recalling each item as one goes.

Use the first-letter method: Acronyms and abbreviations are useful strategies—one can create original acronyms to remember just about anything.

Use "chunking": It is generally easier to remember groups of letters, numbers, or words than to recall each individual item. For example, 1364279805 versus 136-427-9805.

Cluster information by topic: Shopping lists and other information will be easier to remember if it is clustered into groups, such as vegetables, beverages, meats, etc.

Invent rhymes: If they make a catchy rhyme, they'll remember it for a very long time.

Get emotional: Memory can be improved by engaging oneself in what one is trying to remember, creating an emotional reaction.

Test oneself: An excellent way to remember things is to summarize the key points, write them on flashcards, and test oneself with the flashcards.

Write it down: Just the process of writing down information will help one remember it.

When it's on the tip of one's tongue, relax: Becoming tense and anxious makes it more difficult to recall names and other information. Repeating the wrong name often blocks the right one—encourage thinking of other things about the individual instead.

Learn the name well in the first place: Help them pay full attention when they are learning a new name. Have them repeat the name aloud. They should then connect the name to something or someone they know. Encourage them to make a visual image of the person and their new connection with the name. Instruct them to find something in the person's appearance that reminds them of the new name. Ensure that they repeat the name again periodically.

Review names prior to attending a social event: It never hurts to be prepared.

It's OK to forget a name: Help your loved one to not feel stressed or embarrassed if they forget a name. There is nothing wrong in simply saying, "I'm sorry that I can't recall your name. Would you remind me?"

Memory aids can benefit everyone with mild memory problems

Jack sits down at the pottery wheel. He looks up at the instructions that Sara wrote out for him in large letters with a marker.

Step 1: Pick your clay. He looks through several plastic bags until he finds a piece of red clay about the size of a grapefruit.

Jack looks up again. *Step 2: Determine your method—wheel, pinch, coiling, or slab.*

Following the instructions, Jack works throughout the afternoon until, at last, he removes the bowl from the wheel. He smiles as he washes the clay off his hands, satisfied that he is still able to accomplish something.

Everyone with mild memory problems can benefit from memory aids. There are three golden rules for success when using memory aids:

- **Rule 1: Don't delay.** To keep track of things with memory aids, use them promptly. For example, write down appointments immediately and take medications when the reminder alarm goes off.
- **Rule 2: Keep it simple**. Avoid redundancy; simplicity reduces confusion. For example, use one calendar, not four.

• **Rule 3: Make it routine**. Use memory aids all the time, every time. Make a habit of using them, and they will become an automatic part of your daily life.

Here are some of these memory aids that can help your loved one and a brief description of each:

Use an organizer: Organization can help compensate for memory problems when doing many tasks, including paying the bills, balancing the checkbook, and going shopping.

Write out instructions: Many tasks are easy enough to do if one can remember all the steps—the problem is keeping all the steps in mind. Writing out step-by-step instructions provides a simple solution. Use a white board if the instructions are important for today.

Designate a memory table: If your loved one always puts their keys, glasses, phone, and wallet in the same place each day, they will never go missing. For example, use the hall table or a basket by the back door for this purpose. As Benjamin Franklin liked to say, "A place for everything and everything in its place."

Rely on calendars or daily planners: Place the calendar or planner where it will be seen at least daily. Include the five "W"s in each appointment: *When* is the appointment (date and time)? *Who* is the appointment with? *Where* is the location and phone number of the appointment? *What* is the appointment for? *What* should you bring with you to the appointment? You can also use a white board to remind your loved one about important appointments today.

Take advantage of technology: Take advantage of as much technology as your loved one is able to use, such as smartphones with electronic to-do lists, calendars, and alarms.

Keep a notebook: A small notebook kept in one's pocket or purse can be useful to record and retrieve any information.

Make lists: Whether grocery, shopping, or to-do, lists can help your loved one remember what needs to be done.

Use reminder notes: Sticky notes can be put on the door, refrigerator, bathroom mirror, and any other place one can think of to remind one to do something. Just remember to remove the note once the task is done.

ENSURE MEDICATIONS ARE TAKEN CORRECTLY

Taking medications properly is important. With many medications, life-threatening problems can occur if doses are missed or taken twice. If your loved one has been taking their medications on their own for years, it can be tempting to simply let them continue. Perhaps they keep their medication bottles on the nightstand and have been taking them every day before they go to bed. But how would you know if they miss a dose or if they take a dose twice? The reason that keeping medication bottles on a table and taking them at a certain time of day typically fails when one has even very mild dementia is that this system relies on memory. One first must remember to take the medications and then one must remember that the medications have been taken (so that they are not taken again). Luckily, there are many good solutions.

Count the pills

"But, Sara," Jack exclaims, "I don't want a pillbox! I've got a system so I never forget my medications. I have them right here at the breakfast table: medications for cholesterol, blood pressure, and memory."

"But how do you remember to take them each day—and not take them twice?"

"I take my pills when I have breakfast; that's my system."

"Hmm," Sara says, thinking. "What about this: You take each of these medications once a day, right?"

"Yes," Jack says cautiously.

"So, if I count the pills that are in each bottle now, and I recount them next week, there should be seven fewer, right?"

"That makes sense."

"OK, then. If your system works, I promise we'll leave it alone. But
   if it doesn't, can we try a pillbox?"

"You've got yourself a deal."

Sara is counting the pills a week later.

"Dad, you took five from this bottle, so you missed 2 days."

"I missed 2 days?"

"Yes, and from this bottle you took four pills, and from the last one
   you took 10!"

"Oh, so I took too many of those. Well, they all average out!"

"No, they don't, and even if they did, you cannot take medications
   like that. You need to take one pill from each bottle every day.
   Can we try the pillbox now?"

Jack scowls but says reluctantly, "Alright, I'll give it a try."

If your loved one only has mild memory problems and you
think that their old system of taking medications directly from
their bottles is still working, you can easily check and make
sure. Simply count and write down the number of pills that are
in each bottle. Next note how many pills should be taken each
day from each bottle. Return a week later and count the pills
again. Are the correct number of pills in each bottle? If so, then
good; the old system is still working. If not, then a new system
is needed—and needed today!

Have family, friends, or professionals give them their medications

If you (or another family member or friend) are living in or
near their home, one simple solution is for you to give them
their medications. You can use whatever system you wish to
make sure the medications are being taken correctly, but you
may wish to use one of the systems described next. If there are
no family members, friends, or neighbors who can help, a nurse
can be hired to administer the medications, or other professionals can remind your loved one to take them.

Use a pillbox

"OK, Dad," Sara says, "I've put your medications in this pill box for the next 2 weeks. Each day at breakfast time this little alarm will go off."

"An alarm? Why do I need an alarm?"

"So you won't forget to take them."

There are numerous styles of pillboxes available today. A basic pillbox has one compartment for each day of the week and comes in 1-week, 2-week, and 1-month options. There are also pillboxes with two compartments each day (for morning and evening pills) and some with three compartments (for morning, afternoon, and evening medications). They can have a variety of other options, including color-coded compartments, Braille lettering, built-in alarms, display screens, and even communication devices that alert family members when medications are taken. You may want to speak to your loved one's doctor to find the right pillbox for them. Some providers may give you a free pillbox, and some insurance companies will cover its cost.

Once you have a pillbox for your loved one, the next step is to determine how it will be used. Some individuals with *very mild* dementia may be able to fill their pillbox and use it to take their medications correctly by themselves. Individuals with *mild* dementia will generally need you to help them fill their pillbox but then can take the pills on their own. In both of these cases, you should routinely check the pillbox to make sure it is being used correctly. In individuals with *moderate* dementia, you need to both fill the pillbox and supervise them taking their medications. Some families have found success in calling their loved one on the phone and having them take their medications right then and there, while they are on the phone. In this stage of dementia the pillbox is mainly a tool to help you or another caregiver make sure that medications are being administered correctly.

Lastly, pharmacy-filled blister packs are becoming more common and are essentially prefilled pillboxes. This option is ideal because no one has to fill a pillbox and you know the pills are in there correctly. Check to see if your pharmacy has this option available.

USE PICTURES INSTEAD OF WORDS

Pictures are easier to remember than words. Some of our own research found that using pictures for remembering is particularly helpful for individuals with dementia, whose words may begin to disappear due to the damage from their brain disease. You can take advantage of this simple fact by using pictures whenever you want your loved one to remember something, whether it is events on the calendar, a shopping list, or a schedule of who they will be seeing and what they will be doing today.

How do you get the pictures? Most people either find the pictures on the internet or use their smartphone to take the pictures they want. You'll need a printer to print the pictures out. You can also cut pictures out of magazines or newspapers. Use glue or tape to put the pictures into your calendar, daily planner, or wherever you want them.

BE SAFE IN THE KITCHEN

Jack adds another dash of hot sauce as he stirs the beans, carrots, celery, and onions.

"It smells good, Dad," Sara says.

"Just you wait till you taste it!" Jack begins. "I want to thank you for helping me, Sara. The instructions for the pottery, the pillbox, the picture calendar, they're all great. But the best thing is this system for the stove. Now I can make my five-alarm chili—without setting off the smoke alarm!"

> "Yes," Sara says, smiling. "With this motion sensor that turns off the stove if you walk away, and this smoke detector stove shut-off as a backup, you should do fine. But you should try this new microwave I bought you; it's the safest way to cook."

One of the more serious consequences of memory problems is that individuals may leave the stove on, which can result in damage to pots, pans, and sometimes an entire house. We feel strongly that safety measures must be instituted at the first sign of any difficulty using the stove or remembering to turn it off. Which safety measure to institute depends on what the problem using the stove is, how impaired your loved one is, and whether cooking on the stove is something that is important for them. Next we list a number of possible solutions. If you're not sure which is best for your loved one, please consult their doctor.

- *Unplug the stove so that it can't be used. Have them use a micro-wave, toaster, and/or slow cooker instead.* This is an easy solution when the stove is not needed.
- *Take the knobs off the stove so that it can't be used.* If you keep the knobs with you or hidden in the house, this solution has the advantage of allowing you and others to visit and use the stove when you wish to, while still keeping your loved one safe when you are not there.
- *Have an electrician install a switch in a hidden or difficult-to-reach location such that you can use it but your loved one cannot.* This solution also has the same advantage of allowing you and others to visit and use the stove when you wish, while still keeping your loved one safe when you're not there.
- *Install a device with a motion sensor that automatically shuts off the stove.* These devices will turn the stove off after a certain number of minutes (which you can set) if no motion near the stove is detected. Although cumbersome when cooking chili or stew that requires simmering for a long time, this device is ideal for many families.
- *Install a device with a smoke detector that automatically shuts off the stove.* These devices automatically turn off the stove when the

smoke detector alarm sounds. We don't usually recommend the device by itself, but it can be a good backup plan when used with other methods.

- *Combine several of these methods.* For example, if your loved one is usually a reliably safe cook who nevertheless does occasionally walk away and forget that they have something on the stove, install both the motion sensor device and the smoke detector device.

STOP THE SINK OR TUB FROM OVERFLOWING

Although not generally as serious as leaving the stove on, leaving the water running in the tub or sink such that it overflows and floods the house can cause serious damage. There are many solutions to this problem; here are several possibilities:

- *Turn off the water pipe to the sink or tub that is overflowing.* This solution works well if there are several sinks and tubs in the house and only one of them tends to be forgotten and left to overflow.
- *Use a tub alarm.* There are many models available; find the one that works best for your situation.
- *Have a plumber enlarge the overflow drain or decrease the flow of the water such that the tub or sink cannot overflow.* Overflow drains in sinks and tubs are designed to prevent them from overflowing. The problem is that sometimes the flow of water exceeds the capacity of the overflow drain. A plumber can help.

DON'T TELL A PERSON WITH DEMENTIA WHAT NOT TO DO—TELL THEM WHAT THEY SHOULD DO!

"Hello?" Jack answers.

"Dad, it's Sara. There is construction on Main Street, so make sure you go a different way to meet us at the mall."

"OK, thanks."

"So, remember, don't take Main Street."

"I've got it, kid: construction on Main Street."

"Alright, I'll see you in half an hour."

Jack pulls up an hour later.

"Where have you been? Did you get lost?"

"Well, you told me to take Main Street to avoid the construction, but there was construction on Main Street too, so it took a long time."

"Dad, I specifically told you NOT to take Main Street."

"Really? I could have sworn you said that I should take Main Street. Are you sure?"

Sara doesn't respond. She looks at her father with concern and thinks, *I can't believe his memory is this bad.*

One type of false memory that is common in everyone—even those without a memory problem—is believing that an incorrect or untrue statement is actually true. In one study we conducted, we gave healthy older adults and individuals with mild dementia due to Alzheimer's disease a list of statements that were randomly assigned to being either true or false. For example, "It takes 36 coffee beans to make a cup of espresso: True," and "The 53 bus will take you across town: False." Later, we presented the statements again and asked the participants whether each sentence was true or false. Although participants generally found it easy to recall that the true sentences were true, they were highly likely to recall that the false sentences were also true—more than half the time for those with dementia!

The bottom line is that one should rarely tell an individual with dementia what is wrong or false or incorrect, because they will likely end up believing that it is true. Instead, tell them what is correct. Similarly, don't tell a person with dementia what *not* to do, because they might falsely remember that they are supposed to do it! Tell them what they should do.

HABITS AND ROUTINES ARE OFTEN PRESERVED AND CAN BE LEARNED THROUGH REPETITION

Martin uses gentle pressure on each of Nina's hands as she squeezes toothpaste onto her toothbrush and begins to brush her teeth. He guides her, hand over hand, making sure the bristles reach her back teeth.

He has been helping her brush her teeth more independently for the last few months. When he started, she needed full guidance on every step. Now she can do most steps with just a light touch. He knows she may never again be completely independent in her toothbrushing, but he cannot help feeling pride that she is improving each week.

Because they use a different part of the brain than remembering information and events, procedures, habits, routines, and motor skills—such as playing the piano or riding a bike—are relatively unaffected by Alzheimer's disease and most other causes of dementia. Because this type of "procedural memory" or "habit learning" is relatively preserved in dementia, many individuals with mild or even moderate dementia can learn new (and improve old) procedural skills.

Procedural skills and habits are not learned by verbal instruction. They are learned by doing. Another term for this type of memory is "muscle memory." Even though the actual learning is still taking place in the brain, it's helpful to think about the process as muscles learning by practice.

Note that your loved one will not be able to remember instructions. The most effective method is to guide your loved one "hand over hand" without using any words at all. Here are a few examples of activities that could possibly be learned or improved:

- Improve their balance by practicing yoga, tai chi, or a similar activity.
- Improve their dancing ability through classes.
- Improve their backhand on the tennis court through lessons.
- Learn to always put their purse, keys, glasses, wallet, and cellphone in the same place each day.
- Learn a new tune on a musical instrument that they have played for years.
- Learn a simple craft, painting, or drawing well enough to enjoy.
- Find their way to the dining room, bedroom, and bathroom when they move to a new location.
- Improve their activities of daily living such as dressing and toothbrushing.

Not everyone will be able to improve their activities in this way. Everyone begins with different abilities, skills, and talents, and everyone's dementia is also different—even if caused by the same disease. If you try to help your loved one improve a skill and it doesn't work, don't be discouraged. They may still be able to improve a different skill and, even if they cannot, you should feel good that you tried!

ELIMINATE WANDERING

After dinner, Martin begins to do the dishes while Nina heads to the television in the living room.

Half an hour later he walks into the living room. Although the television is on, Nina is not sitting on the couch.

"Honey! Nina! Where are you?" It is as he is looking around the room that he notices it.

"Oh no," he says as his eyes grow wide: The front door is ajar. He rushes over and flings it open.

"Nina!" he yells into the twilight.

He can see no one. He jogs to the end of their walkway. He looks left, right, and left again. Is there a figure disappearing into the distance?

"Nina!" he calls as he jogs toward the figure.

After what seems like a long time, he catches up with the figure.

"Nina! Where are you going?"

"Home," she says.

"Come on, honey, home is back this way." Martin feels his heart thumping against his chest as he watches her shuffle back to their house. *That was close!* he thinks.

We often use the term "wandering" to describe when someone with dementia leaves their home and begins walking somewhere. Wandering may occur for many reasons. The individual with dementia may be trying to get somewhere in the past, such as their childhood home. They may leave the house to go to work, forgetting that they haven't worked for 20 years. Or perhaps they simply want to take a walk around the block and become lost along the way.

Wandering is a very serious problem that can result in disorientation, injury, and death. If your loved one exhibits any type of wandering behavior, such as opening the front door or actually going outside, we recommend that you immediately work to prevent wandering and introduce measures that could be used to track them should they wander out of the house (or a restaurant or shop) despite your best efforts. Here we list a number of methods that can be used to prevent wandering and help return them home safely if they do.

Use visual cues and redirection

Sometimes simple visual cues are effective, such as a red, octagonal "STOP sign" banner that can be placed on a door or across a doorway, providing a visual clue to your loved that they shouldn't go past it. If they are determined to leave the house, sometimes redirecting them to another activity, such as taking a walk around the block with them or giving them a brief ride in the car, can resolve the situation with minimal conflict.

Lock the doors

One simple measure to prevent wandering is to install locks so the doors cannot be easily opened from the inside of the house. However, you need to make sure that you can open the doors quickly in case of a fire. The best locks are those that are fast and easy for you to open but are either out of sight or complicated enough that your loved one will not be able to use them. Often simple sliding locks on the top and bottom of the door are sufficient. Or you could use a latch at eye level that requires two or more steps to unlock. Some childproof locks will also work, depending on the individual and their strength.

Use an alarm

Martin lays a rubber mat with a cord attached in front of the door inside the house and puts their old carpeted doormat on top of it. He then plugs the cord into the wall. He steps on the mat and an alarm rings, which stops as soon as he steps off.

"I know the stop sign didn't work, but do you really need the mat, Pop?" their son asks. "Don't you think the sliders we installed will stop her?"

"Well, I want to know if she's at the door—I don't want her struggling with it for 10 minutes and getting frustrated. And if she finds the sound unpleasant—and who wouldn't!—she may stop approaching the door altogether."

From a simple mechanical bell that will ring when a door is opened to a sophisticated home alarm system, using a method to signal when a door is approached or opened can alert you if your loved one is trying to leave the house. There are also bed alarms that will alert you when your loved one gets up in the middle of the night—which is important if that is a time when they wander. Similarly, there are also chair alarms that tell you when your loved one gets up out of their favorite chair, and motion alarms that can be set to sound when someone is near the door.

Provide supervision

It is a simple thing to say that individuals who could wander should be supervised, but we know it is a much more difficult thing in life to actually do. Nonetheless, if your loved one has shown signs of wandering, we recommend that someone be with them all the time. Use respite care and day programs. Enlist family and friends to spend a few hours with them each week. Speak with others in your care team to help you find solutions. (We'll explain how to build your care team in *Chapter 15.*)

Identification jewelry, tracking devices, and emergency response services

Because wandering is common in dementia and can lead to such serious problems, we recommend that all individuals with dementia wear identification bracelets or other jewelry that includes their name, diagnosis, and emergency number to call. Some programs also allow you to obtain identification jewelry for yourself, which can help to normalize the wearing of such items if you think your loved one may feel stigmatized by it. Search the internet or see the *Further Resources* section at the end of this book for more information.

We know of a few individuals who seem to be magicians at getting out of the house, despite their caregivers' best efforts. There are also individuals who are only in the mild stage of dementia and are not going to wander off but get lost quite frequently. In either of these cases, a tracking device worn on the wrist can be helpful. For individuals who are used to wearing a watch, wearing a tracking device often feels fine and, in fact, there are many electronic watches on the market today that can be used to track your loved one through GPS (global positioning system), cellular, and Wi-Fi signals. Some of these watches are specifically made for this purpose, while others are smart-watches that anyone might purchase. There are also other types of GPS trackers that can be worn on the wrist, around the neck, or attached to clothing. Some trackers allow two-way communication, and other trackers can be easily hooked into the police system so that law enforcement can help with tracking if necessary.

Write a plan for wandering, just in case

When your loved one actually wanders off, it is very difficult to stay calm and think clearly. That's one reason why it is best to write a plan now, just in case it happens. You might want to include the following information in your plan:

- A list of people to call on for help, with their phone numbers
- A dozen recent photographs of your loved one that you can give to police and volunteers
- A dozen copies of their updated medical information that can also be given to police and other emergency personnel
- Areas in your neighborhood that could pose dangers such as busy streets, forests, or bodies of water
- A list of places that you think they might try to get to, whether it is a friend's house, corner store, childhood home, or where they used to work

USE TECHNOLOGY

We live in an age where new technological products, phone applications, and websites are being produced at a dizzying rate. Many of these innovations are being developed with seniors in mind, and many others that are designed for everyone may still be useful for a problem that you and your loved one are dealing with. It never hurts to search the internet for technological solutions to any problem that you are finding challenging to solve.

MAKE PEOPLE AND PLACES
MORE FAMILIAR

"Are you sure, Pop? You really want to give me all the new furniture and take back your old stuff?" their son asks.

"Yes, I'm sure," Martin says as he looks at Nina sitting stiffly on their new sofa. "I want to do anything I can to help your mother feel more at home."

By the end of the day, the old sofa, armchair, and other pieces of furniture are back in Martin and Nina's house.

"So, what do you think, Nina? Do you like having our old furniture back?"

As if responding, Nina settles into the sofa, contented.

As your loved one's memory becomes progressively impaired by dementia, they will usually remember less from the recent past and more from the distant past. They may only recall things from decades earlier—perhaps from their early adult life or even their childhood. For this reason, it is usually comforting for them to be in a place that has some familiar things from the past, such as photographs, art, and other decorations that may have been in the house they grew up in; furniture from that time period; and even music that they enjoyed as young adults. You can work to include some familiar decorations, furniture, and music in their current home.

Similarly, your loved one is more likely to recognize people who look, dress, and wear their hair similarly to how they did in the past, compared with people who look very different today. If your loved one is having difficulty recognizing you (or another family member or close friend), you might try to dress and appear the way you did many years ago—it might help, and there is no harm in trying!

SHADOWING

Does your loved one follow you from room to room and not let you out of their sight? Have you heard of the phrase, "Out of sight, out of mind"? That is literally what is happening here. Because the dementia impairs their ability to form new memories, if your loved one cannot see you, they may not remember where you are, when they have seen you last, or even if you are in the same house. They may think you have been gone for hours when you just used the bathroom for 10 minutes. Particularly if they are having trouble recognizing their home, they may feel anxious if they cannot see you, as you may be the only thing in their world that feels familiar to them. For these reasons they may follow you around, becoming your shadow.

The first thing to note about shadowing is that it isn't a terrible thing. There is nothing wrong with your loved one wanting to be with you. Having said that, there may be times when you have an appointment or just need a little time for yourself. In addition to having someone else spend time with your loved one, other strategies that may work include redirecting them to an activity that they can do on their own, giving them a picture of you that they can look at and keep with them, and having them spend time with a household pet or even a stuffed animal.

DON'T FIGHT FALSE MEMORIES

"Where's James?" Nina asks.

Martin looks up from his book, startled to see her standing over him. "Our son James? James isn't here; he's probably at work."

"I need to get him ready for school."

Martin bites his lip as he thinks about what he should say. *The last time I corrected Nina when she was having a false memory—and I explained to her that she had dementia—all it did was make her cry.* He looks up at her anxious face in front of him. *OK, let's think about the 4Rs: reassure, reconsider, redirect, and relax.*

He stops biting his lip, takes in a breath, and lets it out slowly. Then he puts on a smile and says, "Everything's fine, honey. James had to go to school early, so I drove him this morning. Here," he pauses as he gets up. "Let's take a look at one of our old photo albums of James when he was in school."

He and Nina spend the next 30 minutes smiling and laughing as they go through the old photo album.

Now that wasn't so hard, Martin thinks to himself. *I just need to remember to use the 4Rs all the time.*

We generally expect that when we retrieve a memory it will be accurate. It turns out, however, that memories frequently become distorted, mixed up with other memories, or otherwise confused. Have you ever thought that one of your friends told you something but later realized it was a different friend? Mixing up elements of memories occurs frequently even in healthy individuals, and it is just one cause of false memories.

False memories are more common in dementia. Your loved one's faulty memory may lead them to remember all sorts of things that are not true, such as thinking that they are still working when they retired many years ago, believing that their parents are still alive when they are long since deceased, and recalling that they already took their medication when they did not. They may also confuse things that happened to someone else with things that happened to them—maybe even something that they saw on television!

The best advice we can give if your loved one is having false memories is to not fight them or even try to correct them unless they are distressing. If, after watching a travel program, your loved one thinks that they took a trip to Venice even though they have never been to Italy, don't bother correcting them—let them enjoy the fantasy. If they falsely remember that a family member—now deceased—is going to come pick them up and take them "home," you might want to simply reassure them and redirect them to another activity or topic of conversation.

Sometimes your loved one may mix up memories and become convinced that someone who loves them did something hurtful to them, when it actually isn't true at all. They may become upset when they see the person because of this false memory. In these circumstances the *4Rs* may again be helpful: Reconsider the situation from their point of view, relax as you reassure them that whatever it is isn't true, and then redirect them to another activity or topic. Have the individual who is "accused" of doing the hurtful thing spend time with your loved one doing enjoyable activities. Because emotional memory is relatively preserved in dementia, they may soon develop a good feeling about the person and stop remembering their false memory.

REMINDING THE PERSON WITH DEMENTIA THAT THEY HAVE MEMORY PROBLEMS IS USUALLY NOT HELPFUL

One thing that is tricky about dementia is that people literally have trouble remembering all the times that they forget things. It is for this reason that they often underestimate how impaired their memory is—or they may not remember that they are impaired at all. Similarly, as their memory deteriorates they may completely forget that they have dementia, such that every time they are told they have the disorder, they experience the news as if they are hearing it for the first time.

In general, it isn't useful to remind people that they have dementia—it usually just makes them sad or they may argue with you. We recommend trying to avoid this topic altogether. There are, however, a few times that it may be helpful to point out that they are having a bit of trouble with their memory, such as when you are explaining to them why you are now using a pillbox or have taken the knobs off the stove or are no longer allowing them to drive. In these situations, we usually recommend just reminding them that they have had some trouble managing these activities, rather than reminding them about their specific diagnosis. Having said that, there are some individuals who will be more accepting of help if they are reminded that they have a diagnosis of Alzheimer's disease or dementia. You may need to try out different explanations of why they need help and see which are most effective for your loved one.

SUMMARY

There are many practical things that you can do to help manage your loved one's memory problems. If their dementia is fairly mild, memory strategies and aids can often help. Using a pill-box or another method to ensure that medications are being taken correctly is critical. Pictures are more easily learned than words. Don't tell a person with dementia what not to do; tell them what they should do. Habits and routines are generally preserved in dementia, and new ones can be learned. Use methods to make sure the stove is not left on and the water is not left running. Work to eliminate wandering and write a plan in case it occurs. Take advantage of technological solutions to memory problems. Use reminders of the past to make your loved one feel more at home. Don't fight false memories. Lastly, reminding your loved one that they have memory problems is rarely helpful.

Let's consider some examples to illustrate what we learned in this chapter.

- *He has asked me what we are doing today 10 times in the last hour. What can I do about this?*
  - There are several strategies that may help. You can provide him with a calendar with pictures of what he will do each day and, using habit, teach him to look at the calendar whenever he asks.

Or you might simply redirect him to an activity that will keep him occupied.

- *I came home from the hairdresser the other day and, when I said "Hello," he asked me who I was and what I was doing in his house. At first I thought he was joking, but he really didn't recognize me. How can I help him to recognize me?*

  - The first thing to do is to relax, and remember it's the dementia that is causing the problem. Confirm that he recognizes you in old pictures. If you look more similar to how you appeared in the old pictures—which may require a change in hairstyle or clothing—he is more likely to recognize you.

- *This is the second time that I have found him wandering three blocks from the house. What should I do?*

  - Use the *ABCs of Behavior Change* method in *Chapter 4* to understand the antecedents to wandering. Put stop signs and locks on the door. Consider an alarm that will sound if he approaches or opens the door. Use identification jewelry and programs to help return him safely if he is found wandering. Consider tracking devices or providing him with supervision all the time. Write a plan for what you will do in case you cannot find him quickly.

- *Now my mother is having false memories—she tells me she spoke to her parents last night, but they've been dead for 30 years! Should I correct her and tell her she's wrong?*

  - No. Unless there is some reason to correct her, it's best to just ignore the false memory and redirect her to another activity or topic of conversation.

6

How to manage language problems

In this chapter we will consider some of the reasons that speaking and comprehending language can break down in aging and dementia—why there is sometimes difficulty translating sound into meaning and turning meaning into sounds and grammatical sentences. We will begin by reviewing why problems with language occur in dementia, and then turn to various ways to improve difficulties in hearing, understanding, and speaking.

THE BRAIN CONVERTS SOUNDS INTO WORDS, SENTENCES, AND MEANING

To understand speech, we first need to hear the word correctly. Next, the outer and lower part of the temporal lobe, just behind your eyes, deciphers the sounds of the word and connects those sounds to its meaning. This part of the brain understands not only words but also who and what people and things are, including how you might categorize them. There is a gradient of knowledge such that people (Mary, friend from school; John, colleague at work; Susan, my sister) are in the front, animals (poodle, pet; lion, zoo animal; chicken, farm animal) are in the middle, and human-made objects (desk, office furniture;

baseball bat, sports equipment; hairbrush, morning routine) are in the back. This stored knowledge forms the basis of the vocabulary we draw from when we speak. Names of the people and objects are stored in this part of the brain on the left, whereas the analogous area on the right stores what qualities things have—such as whether they are large or small, light or heavy, hard or soft. So, if the temporal lobes are not working correctly, there will be impairment in both understanding and producing language.

Broca's area, in the frontal lobe of the brain, coordinates the activity of speaking. First, the idea or content we wish to express is chosen. Second, a brain network finds the right words to say the content. Lastly, the words are put into grammatical sentences and it's all converted into sounds. When Broca's area is not working correctly, there will be difficulty speaking and finding words.

WORD-FINDING DIFFICULTY IS COMMON IN ALL STAGES OF DEMENTIA

In normal aging there is often difficulty coming up with names of people, places, books, movies, and other proper nouns, whereas even in mild dementia there may also be difficulty coming up with ordinary, common nouns for everyday things. These difficulties may manifest as the wrong or less precise term being used (for example, flower for rose, table for desk) or, more commonly, simply by pauses in sentences when the word is searched for. Friends and families often get used to jumping in during these pauses to provide the missing word.

It can take effort, even for healthy individuals, to find the right word. That's why when an individual is tired or sick or otherwise not at their best it can be particularly hard to find the correct word—especially when dementia has damaged the language system.

THE MEANING OF WORDS AND OBJECTS CAN DETERIORATE IN DEMENTIA

"Now, Nina, what are you doing with that fork?" Martin asks.

Nina is using a plastic fork in her hair as if it were a comb.

"There's a comb right here, honey," Martin says as he picks up a plastic comb from the coffee table. "Why don't you try this instead?"

Nina pauses, looks at the comb, and resumes using the fork.

Martin slowly shakes his head as he thinks, *At first she couldn't find the words for things like fork and comb, but now she doesn't seem to know one from the other.*

A few minutes later Nina is peering around the edges of the television, looking from side to side.

"Honey, there are no knobs on this TV," Martin says. "Come here and use this remote if you want to change the channel." Nina looks at the remote in Martin's hand as if she's never seen one before. *I think she's forgotten what a remote control is,* Martin thinks, *or even that TVs now have remotes and not knobs.*

When dementia affects the language system in the brain, knowledge of people and objects may become lost. When this loss occurs, not only is there difficulty searching for the name of an object, but there is also difficulty in understanding what the object is, what qualities it has, and what it is used for. This loss of object knowledge generally occurs in the moderate or severe dementia stages.

HEARING AIDS CAN HELP

Approximately one-third of people between the ages of 65 and 75 have hearing loss, as do nearly half of those over the age of 75. If your loved one hasn't had their hearing tested recently, set up an evaluation through their doctor. If they already have a hearing aid, make sure that it is working well for them. Look at the new models and see if any would work better than their current one. Some hearing aids now use Bluetooth technology to link directly to a cellular phone, dramatically improving hearing on the telephone.

If your loved one is resistant to wearing hearing aids, talk to them about it. Some people don't like the way they look or the stigma associated with wearing them. Explain to them that there are some hearing aids that are barely noticeable. Other people feel that they can hear just fine without them— but only because everyone else is speaking at the top of their voice! Explain to your loved one that the hearing aids are not just for their benefit, but also for the benefit of the people around them.

HELP THOSE WITH HEARING LOSS UNDERSTAND YOU

There are many things that you can do to help your loved one with hearing loss understand what you are saying.

- Find a quiet place to talk with little background noise. For example, restaurants vary in how much ambient noise is present. At social events you may want to move to a quiet corner or even another room to talk.
- Make sure only one person speaks at a time.
- Face your loved one and maintain good eye contact.
- Speak slowly and clearly.
- Speak a bit louder than normal, but don't shout.
- Don't eat or chew gum while talking.
- Repeat yourself if necessary, using different words to make the same point. Some words may be easier to hear and understand than others.

READING AND WRITING MAY BE BENEFICIAL FOR THOSE WHO HAVE MILD DEMENTIA

If your loved one has only mild dementia and they have great difficulty hearing, it may be easier for you to write down what you wish to tell them and have them read it, rather than yelling at them (or into the telephone). Many older adults find reading a letter or an email much easier than communicating by phone.

Similarly, if your loved one has mild dementia and slurred speech due to strokes or other problems that impair the movement of their lips, mouth, tongue, and vocal cords, they may be able to communicate more effectively by writing or typing than speaking.

SPEECH THERAPY MAY BE HELPFUL IN MILD DEMENTIA

Speech therapy is frequently recommended to help individuals who have trouble with articulation following a stroke, but it may also be helpful to those with speech problems due to some causes of mild dementia, particularly if the dementia affects speech or is due to strokes. (See *Chapter 3*, where vascular dementia and the non-fluent/agrammatic variant of primary progressive aphasia are discussed.) Speech therapists will typically meet with your loved one once a week for a series of weeks or months, depending on their progress and insurance coverage. Note that it is critical that you (or another member of the care team) accompany them to the appointment so that you will know what they need to practice. Just like learning a musical instrument or any other skill, it is essential that they practice their assigned speech exercises daily. Your encouragement and practicing with them will help the speech therapy be successful.

USE PICTURES FOR COMPREHENSION AND COMMUNICATION

Pictures can overcome many language problems. If your loved one is having difficulty finding words or pronouncing them clearly, they may be able to point to a picture of what they want. Pictures can be particularly useful when there are a relatively small number of choices, such as items on a menu, shows on television, exercises one might do, or outings one might go on. Make a page on paper or the computer for each topic of the items your loved one can choose from. They can then simply point to the entrée or show or other item that they desire. There are also many smartphone and tablet applications that can be used for this type of picture-based communication. Most of these applications will come with pictures of basic items such as toilet, shower, toothbrush, shirt, salad, etc., and most will also allow you to insert your own pictures from the internet or your smartphone camera. Because the majority of these applications are designed for tablets, an internet search for "tablet apps for communication" will be a good place to start to find an appropriate application for your loved one. Note that you can also use pictures in a calendar or daily planner to show the relevant activities and people for that day.

USE NONLINGUISTIC AND NONVERBAL COMMUNICATION

"OK, honey," Martin says as he opens the car door. "We're here! Let's give this swim a try."

Nina doesn't move. Martin leans forward to unbuckle her seatbelt and quickly backs off as she begins to strike out with her fists.

Oh no, Martin says to himself as the color drains from his face, *not again.* He begins to feel anxious as Nina starts to tap on the dashboard. *Keep yourself together, Martin. Now is not the time to panic. If she doesn't understand your words, show her what you mean. And show her how much you love her.*

"Come on, Nina, we're going swimming—look, I'll show you," Martin says as he puts his head down and begins to expertly do the crawl stroke with his arms. He stops for a minute, smiles at her, rubs her back, and then pretends to dive into a pool before miming the breaststroke.

Nina is suddenly trying to get out of the car, fighting against the seatbelt.

"Hold on, girl, hold on. Just let me get your seatbelt off. I knew you wanted to go swimming," Martin says, smiling.

Have you ever tried to communicate with someone when you don't know their language? You probably used your hands, gestures, body language, facial expression, and tone of voice to get your point across. You can use all of these methods to communicate with your loved one if they are having difficulty understanding language. A good way to practice is to try to communicate your meaning without speaking at all. When you are with your loved one, however, we generally recommend that you both say what you are trying to communicate and show them with your hands, body, and tone of voice.

VIDEO PHONES MAY BE BENEFICIAL

Because nonverbal communication becomes more important in dementia, communicating with your loved one using a video phone may be better than an ordinary audio phone (whether it is a cellular phone or a landline). With a video phone, gestures, body language, and facial expression can be seen by both parties, providing important cues that can help you and your loved one understand each other even when language itself has broken down. All smartphones allow video communication either through their own internal application or a third-party application. There are also standalone video phones you can purchase.

Some of these standalone phones are designed with older adults in mind and may offer features such as automatic answering when a friend or family member calls, and turning to follow people if they are moving around the room.

EMOTIONAL COMMUNICATION IS GENERALLY PRESERVED IN DEMENTIA

It is worth emphasizing that emotional aspects of communication are often preserved well into the moderate and severe stages of dementia. Your loved one will likely detect and respond to your tone of voice, facial expression, body language, and gestures. So, it is important to be gentle in your touch, show love and reassurance on your face, and express openness with your body language. When they do something that makes you angry or annoyed, remember that it is the dementia—not them—that is the problem. Try not to cross your arms and scowl. Keep your arms open and put a smile on your face. That's usually the fastest way to diffuse the situation.

SUMMARY

Although language may become impaired by dementia, communication with your loved one is still possible. Speak clearly and slowly in a quiet environment. Help them obtain hearing aids, if needed. Reading and writing may be beneficial for those who have hearing or speech problems and mild dementia. Speech therapy may also benefit those with mild dementia and trouble talking. Pictures can often compensate for a variety of comprehension and communication problems. Gestures, body language, facial expression, tone of voice, and other nonlinguistic and nonverbal communication can be useful, both in person and over a video phone. Lastly, remember that emotional communication is often preserved in dementia.

Let's consider some examples to illustrate what we learned in this chapter.

- *My father knows what he wants to say but cannot get the words out. He's becoming more and more frustrated. What can I do to help?*
  - Try using pictures on either paper or a tablet application to help him communicate. Create a different page for each category, such as places, foods, and enjoyable activities. He can then point to what he wants.
- *I keep talking to my wife but it's clear she doesn't understand me. How can I get through to her?*
  - Nonlinguistic and nonverbal communication may help. Try using your hands, gestures, body language, facial expression, and tone of voice to communicate. You can also use pictures.
- *I try to check in with my grandmother once a week by calling her, but even with her hearing aids she has trouble understanding me on the phone. What should I do?*
  - Make sure that her hearing aids are functioning properly and see if there is a newer model that might work even better (such as one that will connect directly to her phone via Bluetooth). If she is able to read, consider writing her a letter or an email to tell her what you have been up to or other information you wish to communicate. Lastly, a video phone may provide improved communication, and seeing your grandmother will help you know how she is doing.
- *I know he's not trying to make a mess, but I cannot help being upset when he does. Even though I don't criticize him with words, I'm sure it shows on my face, and he often starts to cry.*
  - Because emotional communication is relatively preserved in dementia when comprehension of spoken language has deteriorated, he will likely pick up on your mood by your tone of voice, facial expression, and body language. Remember that he's doing as well as he can, think of the *4Rs* (*Chapter 4*), reassure him that everything is alright, and smile. Just the act of smiling may also help lift your mood, despite the mess.

7

How to manage vision problems

In this chapter we will discuss how vision can be disrupted by dementia, leading to everything from difficulty seeing to hallucinations. We will begin by reviewing how eye problems, although not caused by dementia, can disrupt vision, which may greatly impair function. We will then discuss a number of ways to improve visual function in individuals with dementia.

START WITH AN EYE EXAMINATION

Eye problems are the most common cause of visual difficulties in older adults, whether or not they have dementia. Make sure that your loved one sees an eye doctor regularly. The eye doctor can determine if they need new glasses and can check to make sure the glasses made by the optician were done correctly. A standard eye exam will also look for cataracts—another common cause of poor vision—as well as other treatable eye diseases, such as glaucoma and macular degeneration.

ENSURE ADEQUATE LIGHTING

It will be difficult to see if there isn't adequate light—an obvious statement but worth emphasizing. Reassess the lighting both inside and outside your loved one's home, particularly stairs, basements, outdoor walkways, and areas with steps. Make sure the color of light switch panels contrasts with the wall color so that switches can be easily seen. For areas where the lamp or light switch may be difficult to access or on the far side of the room, consider using motion sensors that turn on lights when one enters. Replace old lightbulbs with new fluorescent, light-emitting diode (LED), or halogen bulbs that can give off more light with the same or lower wattage.

INCREASE VISUAL CUES AND CONTRAST

If increasing the amount of light alone isn't adequate or possible, increase visual cues and contrast, such as making it easier to see steps that might have otherwise blended into the background. A coat of paint or strip of brightly colored or fluorescent tape at the edge of each step can increase their visibility—just make sure that the tape is firmly affixed to the step so that it does not become a tripping hazard!

In moderate to severe dementia, there may be difficulty distinguishing items from their visual background when the shades of colors are similar. Few of us would experience difficulty seeing a skinless breast of chicken, fillet of cod, white rice, mashed potatoes, scrambled egg whites, or a slice of white bread on a white plate, but a person with dementia just might! One study found that individuals with dementia living in nursing homes ate more food at each meal when the plates were changed from white to a color (such as red) that contrasted with the color of their food (mostly white). If your loved one is losing weight and not eating all the food on their plate, try increasing the contrast by changing the color of the plate and see if it helps.

ADJUST FOR DIFFICULTY SEEING OR PAYING ATTENTION ON ONE SIDE

One strange but not uncommon problem that may occur is when individuals with dementia do not see things on one side of the world, usually the left. One way to compensate for this problem is to try to keep things on their "good side." Put food on the right side of their plate, set out clothes on the right side of their bed, and so on. If you are out at a restaurant and they only eat food on the right side of their plate, turn the plate around so they'll notice the uneaten food. There are, of course, many things that cannot be moved to their "good side," and thus some activities (such as driving) will need to be stopped.

INCREASE THE SIZE OF NUMBERS AND LETTERS

Your loved one may be able to read and tell time but they may have difficulty seeing the small print in books and newspapers or the small numbers on watches and clocks. Find telephones, clocks, and watches with large numbers. Most libraries have collections of books and newspapers in large print. If not too complicated for them, computers and tablets also allow for letters to be adjusted to virtually any size. Similarly, when writing notes for your loved one, use large letters and write with black felt-tip markers on white paper.

USE ELECTRONIC MAPS AND NAVIGATION SYSTEMS WITH AUDIO DIRECTIONS

"I thought you told me you didn't like using a GPS device," Jack's friend says.
"This isn't a GPS—this is Dick Tracy's watch!" Jack responds.

"Dick Tracy? The comic book detective stories we read as kids?"

"Yes! Look here," Jack says, raising his new wristwatch to his mouth. A tone chimes, and he says, "Directions to home."

"Getting directions to home," the electronic voice in the watch says. "Head northeast on Main Street, then turn left."

"Wow," his friend says, "that's amazing!"

"Not only that, if I do get lost, I can call my daughter with it. Look," Jack says as he again raises the watch to his mouth. "Call Sara," he says after the chime.

When poor vision obscures landmarks, it is easy to get lost whether one is driving or walking. Visual problems may also make reading paper and electronic maps and GPS devices difficult. If visual difficulties are the major reason that your loved one is becoming lost, try an electronic smartphone map application or GPS navigation system with a clear audio output. There are even smartwatches that can provide step-by-step audio directions. Just make sure that the system is helpful and not merely distracting—the last thing you want to do is to cause an accident! You should also consider one of the many tracking devices available in case your loved one does become lost, despite your best efforts.

ILLUSIONS OCCUR WHEN THERE ARE MISPERCEPTIONS

Have you ever looked at something quickly and thought it might be a person or an animal, and then you look more closely and you realize it was something else, perhaps a tree or a bush? If so, you've experienced an illusion. We use the term *illusion* when you are perceiving something that is there, but you don't perceive it correctly, and so you make a mistake as to what it is. Illusions are common when vision is poor. Note that illusions are different from hallucinations. As we will discuss later in the chapter, hallucinations occur when you see something even though there is nothing there.

REDUCE THE IMPACT OF HALLUCINATIONS

"Papa?"

Martin opens his eyes and peers into the darkness. As he feared, Nina is again talking to the empty corner of their bedroom.

"What's wrong, Papa?"

"Nina, honey, come back to bed. There's nobody there." She doesn't move, and he clicks on the light. He sees her squint as she stares into the corner.

Sighing, Martin gets out of bed and steps over to her. He rubs her back and says in a reassuring voice, "Everything is OK. Your father isn't here; it's just you and me. Let's go to the bathroom now that you're up."

Nina continues to stare into the corner. He takes her hand and begins to gently pull her toward the bathroom. She resists, standing her ground. He tugs again and she pulls her hand away. "Papa?" she says again.

Martin reconsiders the hallucinations from her perspective. *She clearly thinks she is seeing her father. But it is not upsetting her, so I guess there's no harm in letting her talk to the corner.*

He thinks about how he can redirect her to another activity. "Nina, would you like to see some pictures of your father?" She slowly turns her head, looks at him for a moment, and then stares back into the corner.

He takes in a deep breath and relaxes. *Everything is fine*, he thinks. *It doesn't matter that she is talking to the corner at 3 in the morning.* He walks to the living room, pulls down an old photo album from the bookcase, and brings it to her. "Look, Nina, here are some pictures of your Papa."

Within a few minutes, Nina is sitting on the bed with him, happily looking through the old album. Ten minutes later they have gone to the bathroom and are back in bed.

Martin smiles to himself as he returns to sleep.

Are you concerned that your loved one is hallucinating? First, determine if they are true hallucinations, not illusions or false memories. In true hallucinations you can observe your loved one actively interacting with a person, animal, or object that is not there. Illusions—misperceptions of things that actually are there—are best dealt with by improved vision, whether through better lighting, new eyeglasses, or getting closer to the misperceived object. Next determine if they are false memories. Did your loved one actually see their long-dead mother in your presence, or did they simply tell you that they saw her last night? If the latter, it is much more likely to be a false memory than a hallucination.

For true hallucinations we recommend the *4Rs—reassure, reconsider, redirect,* and *relax* (see *Chapter 4*):

- *Reassure* them that everything is fine, making calm, reality-based statements such as, "Everything is alright; no one is really there."
- *Reconsider* the hallucinations from their perspective. Are they upset by them? The vast majority of individuals with dementia who experience hallucinations are not upset by them—it is mainly their family who find the hallucinations distressing. If this is the case for you, please note that although we certainly want your loved one to be interacting with the real world, many hallucinations are harmless and so there is no need to have them go away completely. If, on the other hand, your loved one finds the hallucinations upsetting or threatening, it then becomes much more important to deal with them.
- *Redirect* them to pleasant activities that will distract them from the hallucinations, such as looking through old photo albums, having a snack, or going for a walk or a drive. Because hallucinations may be associated with a specific place, this last option often works best.
- *Relax*, and remember that our goal is to reduce the amount of time they are hallucinating and to make the hallucinations less threatening. We may not be able to eliminate hallucinations completely, but we can almost always lessen their frequency and impact.

Lastly, there are several classes of medications that can reduce hallucinations and their impact, as we will discuss in *Step 3*.

WHAT TO DO WHEN YOU ARE A STRANGER OR IMPOSTER

Martin senses something is wrong as he and Nina sit down for dinner.

"You're not him," she says. "You're not the *real* Martin."

"I am, honey," he says *reassuringly*. "Maybe you've forgotten how old I've become—how old we've both become—but I really am Martin."

She looks at him suspiciously.

"Here, have some broccoli and chicken," he says, trying to *redirect* her toward dinner as he puts some of each on her plate.

"You're not him," she repeats. "Get out of my house."

He knows that this is just part of her dementia but he cannot stop the tears from coming. He tries to *relax* as he thinks of what he should do. *Well, why not give it a try?*

"OK, Nina, I'll go," he says, wiping his tears. "I'll go out and if I find the real Martin, I'll send him to you."

He puts on his hat and coat and steps out into the evening air, shutting the door behind him. He feels himself relax as he strolls back and forth in front of his house. After about 5 minutes he returns, opening the door noisily.

"Honey, I'm home," Martin calls from the foyer toward the kitchen, just the way he did a thousand times before when he came home from work.

"Martin," he hears her soft voice in reply, "is that you?"

"Yes, honey," he says, as he thinks to himself, *Well, I might as well play the part.* "I'm so sorry that I had to work late at the office. What's for dinner?" he says as he walks into the kitchen.

Nina doesn't respond but is looking at him with recognition in her eyes.

"Oh, chicken and broccoli; doesn't that looks great!"

Some of the most distressing and difficult symptoms are when your loved one does not recognize you, thinks you are someone else, or believes that you have been replaced by an imposter. Here we will discuss three strategies for dealing with these types of symptoms: using the *4Rs*, increasing visual cues, and using auditory cues. Medications can sometimes help; we will discuss these in *Step 3*.

Although the *4Rs* are useful in most situations, they can be particularly useful in this one.

- *Reassure* your loved one with gentle statements such as, "I know I look old enough to be your father, but I'm really George, your husband," or "I understand that I may look a bit different than when I was younger, but I'm not an imposter—I'm your husband, the real George."
- *Reconsider* how you would feel if you didn't recognize the person who says they are your spouse or child. Keeping this reconsideration in mind, realize that if your truthful reassurance isn't helping, you will need to change your reassuring statements to general ones such as, "Everything's alright; you're doing fine."
- *Redirect* your loved one to pleasant activities that might help them recognize you, such as looking through photo albums or doing something that you usually did with them, whether it is singing, dancing, walking, cooking, or working on jigsaw puzzles. These activities will also help to distract them so they will not focus on who you are.
- Lastly, *relax* and recognize that, despite your best efforts, their vision or memory may have deteriorated to the point that they are simply unable to recognize you. You can, however, still enjoy the time you spend together.

Sometimes the difficulty in recognizing you is due to the fact that you look different now compared to how you looked before—before you had gray hair, for example. It may be that the image they are seeing of you now, with gray hair, is actually a better match for their representation of their father, and so when they see you they think you are their father. This error would be particularly likely if, because of their memory problems, they think they are young and don't yet have a spouse or children. For this reason, if it is possible you may consider changing your hairstyle, hair color, or clothing back to the way it was many years ago, which may help your loved one recognize you.

Lastly, sometimes your loved one may think you are someone else when they see you, but they may still recognize you from your voice. For this reason, when they believe you are someone else, it may be beneficial to make a clear show of leaving the house, wait 5 to 15 minutes, and then call either on the phone or just with your voice through the door, and come back in. If you are successful, you may hear an interesting story from them about when a stranger, imposter, or some other person came to the house and pretended that they were you—when, of course, it was really you all along!

WHEN VISUAL SYMPTOMS ARE THE FIRST AND MOST PROMINENT PROBLEM

Lastly, some individuals with dementia have visual problems as their most prominent symptom, while their other cognitive functions, such as memory, language, and behavior, are more or less intact. If this description sounds like your loved one, you may have heard the term *posterior cortical atrophy*. Posterior cortical atrophy is not a disease in itself but is a useful way to describe individuals with dementia who have these types of visual problems as their most prominent symptoms. The name comes from the fact that it is the back or posterior part of the brain that is most affected.

SUMMARY

Whether caused by dementia or an eye disease, problems with vision can disrupt your loved one's function, create hallucinations, and even lead them to think you are an imposter. There are, however, many things you can do to help. Start with an eye examination to make sure their eyeglasses prescription is correct and to look for treatable diseases. Ensure adequate lighting in and around their home and increase visual cues in potentially hazardous areas, such as stairs. Adjust for difficulty seeing or paying attention on one side. Increase visual contrast and size of numbers and letters for their daily activities. Use navigation systems with audible directions. Reduce the impact of hallucinations. Lastly, manage difficulties when your loved one does not recognize you, thinks you are someone else, or believes that you have been replaced by an imposter.

Let's consider some examples to illustrate what we learned in this chapter.

- *My wife is getting lost all the time. I know her vision isn't very good. What can I do to help her?*
  - First, make sure she sees an eye doctor, obtains new glasses if needed, and has any eye diseases treated. If the dementia is very mild, an electronic navigation system with audio directions may prevent her from getting lost whether she is driving or walking. Just make sure that the system is helpful and not distracting— the last thing you want to do is to cause an accident!
- *OK, so we put my father through the cataract surgery and got him new glasses, but he still can't seem to see very well, particularly on the left side. What should we do?*
  - Many individuals with dementia have difficulty seeing things on one side, usually the left, because of how the dementia affects their brain. Try to keep food, clothing, and other items on his "good side." Keep in mind that activities requiring good vision on both sides—such as driving—will need to be stopped.

- *My husband saw his mother last night in our bedroom. I know it was a true hallucination because it happened in front of me. What should I do?*
  - Use the *4Rs*—*reassure* him that everything is alright, *reconsider* the hallucinations from his perspective, *redirect* him to activities that will distract him, and *relax*, remembering that although his hallucinations may be upsetting to you, they may not be upsetting to him. Note that the goal in managing hallucinations is not necessarily to eliminate them, but to reduce their frequency and impact.
- *Half the time my wife thinks I'm her father or her brother, and the other half she recognizes me—but doesn't think I'm the real me! What can I do?*
  - Start with the *4Rs*—*reassure* her that you are her husband, *reconsider* your actions in light of her thinking you are someone else, *redirect* her to activities that may help her recognize you, and finally *relax*, recognizing that due to the dementia, she may not be able to recognize you, despite your efforts. You can also try to make your visual appearance more similar to how it was years ago and to see if she can recognize your voice, which may help her to recognize the rest of you.

8

How to manage emotional problems

Dementia may cause many emotions in your loved one, including frustration, depression, anxiety, and sometimes excessive crying or laughing. Although emotions are not problems themselves, how your loved one is feeling is important. Unrecognized and untreated emotions may lead to behavioral problems and diminished function. In this chapter we will explain why dementia may lead to emotional problems and how you can manage them. As you are reading, you may find yourself thinking that some of the explanations and advice given in this chapter would be applicable to you as well; that is intentional. We'll continue discussing how you can deal with your own emotions, like depression and anxiety, in *Chapter 14*.

DEPRESSION AND ANXIETY ARE COMMON IN DEMENTIA

Over the past month, Sara has become increasingly worried that her father is depressed.

"Dad, I was wondering," Sara begins, "how are you spending your time now that you're no longer working at the pottery shop or playing hockey with your friends?"

"Oh, I fix myself breakfast, watch some TV, then make lunch, and maybe take a naaaap," Jack says, yawning into the phone, "like the one you woke me up from."

Sara pauses before responding, "Dad, you sound a bit depressed."

"Well, I confess that it's hard when half your friends have died, the other half can't do much, and—even with all your help—I'm still struggling to do simple things," Jack says sadly. "I'm going to go now and finish my nap. I'll talk to you later, Sara."

Hmm . . . Dad really sounds sad, Sara thinks, with a catch in her throat.

It is understandable that many people feel sad or anxious when they receive the diagnosis of Alzheimer's disease or another dementia. In addition, dementia can affect your loved one's emotions by directly damaging different parts of the brain. For these reasons, depression and anxiety are common in dementia.

Depression

When sadness lasts for an extended period of time (2 weeks or longer) and impairs functioning, we typically call it *depression*. Depression is not normal and is not to be expected just because your loved one is older and has dementia. Depression can sometimes be difficult to differentiate from dementia, so an evaluation by a physician or neuropsychologist may be needed to know, for example, whether dementia has caused depression or depression has led to difficulties with thinking and memory.

Common symptoms of depression are as follows:

- Feelings of sadness
- Feelings of worthlessness or guilt
- Fixating on past failures
- Being tearful
- Irritability or frustration, even over small matters
- Memory difficulties
- Trouble concentrating

- Sleep difficulties
- Daytime fatigue and lack of energy
- Changes in appetite
- Often wanting to stay at home
- Physical slowing
- Physical aches or pain
- Loss of interest in activities
- Loss of interest in sex
- Loss of interest in living
- Hopelessness about the future
- Frequent thoughts of death

Anxiety

Anxiety typically presents with nervousness and worry, but it can also produce many physical symptoms (see the following list). Understandably, sometimes symptoms of anxiety are attributed to medical problems. On the other hand, many of these symptoms could indicate a very serious medical problem, such as a heart attack. If your loved one is having any of these symptoms, it is important that they see their doctor to look for medical causes, such as heart disease. But if the doctor has ruled out all of the medical problems that could be causing their symptoms, it may be that they have anxiety.

Common symptoms of anxiety are as follows:

- Feeling nervous, restless, or tense
- A sense of impending danger, panic, or doom
- Feeling one's heart beat (palpitations)
- Breathing rapidly
- Sweating
- Trembling
- Feeling weak or tired
- Trouble concentrating
- Trouble thinking about other things
- Stomach or bowel problems
- Difficulty controlling anxious feelings
- Avoiding things that trigger the anxiety

CRYING OR LAUGHING TOO EASILY OR INAPPROPRIATELY MAY OCCUR IN DEMENTIA

Are you worried that your loved one is depressed because they cry spontaneously or with little provocation? Are there times when they laugh when nothing is funny or when it's not socially appropriate to do so? If you see either of these patterns in your loved one, it is worth considering whether these behaviors may be due to the dementia. Doctors often refer to this condition as *pseudobulbar affect* or *pathological laughing and crying*.

If your loved one is crying frequently, they may, of course, be depressed. But don't assume that they are—ask them how they are feeling. If they tell you they are feeling sad and that's why they are crying, then you know they are depressed. If, on the other hand, they tell you they are not sad and they don't know why they are crying, it may be that the damage to the brain from the dementia has made it difficult for them to control their tears. Similarly, spontaneous, exaggerated, or inappropriate laughing could be due to your loved one thinking that something is very funny, or it could be that they cannot control their laughter even when they don't think that anything is funny. Asking them is the best way to sort it out—which is important, because the treatment will depend on the cause, as we will see in *Step 3*.

DEPRESSION AND ANXIETY MAY BE DUE TO DECLINING ABILITIES

One cause of depression and anxiety in dementia—particularly early in the disease—is the normal reaction that any of us would have if it became difficult to carry out daily or enjoyable activities. Frustration at not being able to complete a task can lead to irritability. Mood can also be affected. Worry about how one will be able to manage in the future can lead to depression and anxiety. And the combination of all these emotions plus the impairments in function can lead our loved ones to stop participating because the activities are too difficult, too frustrating, or too depressing—because failing at the activity emphasizes how impaired they really are.

Improve abilities

For these reasons, the first thing to try is to improve their abilities. Sometimes just a small improvement will enable them to resume the activities that are important to them, whether it is working in the garden, knitting clothes for their grandchildren, or ordering food in a restaurant. In *Chapters 5, 6,* and *7* we reviewed ways that memory, language, and visual function can be improved. Use these *Step 2* methods along with those in *Chapter 11* to improve your loved one's abilities. We'll also discuss medications that can improve your loved one's abilities in *Step 3.*

Adjust the task

"Dad, how come you're not making your favorite chili?" Sara asks. "You can use the microwave I bought you."

"That chili recipe is too complicated," Jack responds glumly. "It's *another* thing I can't do. And I certainly can't figure out this new microwave. Look at all the buttons—there must be 30 of them!"

Sara wanted the microwave to be a replacement for the stovetop and oven, so she purchased one with all the features. "Hmm, I see what you mean," she says, looking at it. "Well, I could use a new microwave. Why don't I take this one, and we can go shopping for another."

"What about this one, Dad?" Sara asks at the appliance store.

Jack looks at the microwave, which has just two knobs and no buttons. "Hey, this top knob is just like on the stove—low, medium, and high. And the bottom knob is a timer. Now this is a good one for me!"

Walking to the car, Sara asks, "Dad, how about if I come over for dinner and you can try out your new microwave by making chili with your famous recipe?"

"Well," Jack says uncomfortably, "that's a complex recipe ..."

"I'll help you. We'll get the ingredients on the way home."

Sara sets the ingredients on the kitchen counter in the correct order and puts a little sticky note that says how much of each is needed. With this little bit of help, Jack is able to follow the recipe, put the chili into the microwave, and set the power level and the timer appropriately.

Ding!

"It's ready!" Jack says as he ladles chili into two bowls.

"Good chili, Dad!"

"Thanks, Sara," Jack says with a smile, "and thanks so much for getting me this 'old-person' microwave and setting up the ingredients. I'm going to leave these sticky notes here so I'll always be ready to make my chili recipe."

Try reducing the difficulty of the task your loved one is trying to do. If they can do the simplified task, it may help them to feel better about themselves and less depressed. For example, by helping them get set up in the garden with the tools, seeds, plantings, and other things they will need, you've just turned a very complicated organizational task into a more straightforward one. To aid cooking, set up the ingredients and stay with them during the potentially hazardous parts, such as using the oven and stovetop.

Note that there are certainly some activities that may be either too difficult or hazardous for your loved one to continue participating in, such as playing bridge, using power tools, or driving. In these cases, think of the *4Rs* (*Chapter 4*) and *redirect* them to activities that they can participate in.

TREAT DEPRESSION AND ANXIETY

You may find that your loved one is struggling with depression or anxiety despite your best efforts at increasing their abilities and reducing their difficulties. The good news is that, working with their doctor, you can do many things to improve their mood.

If they are anxious about their memory loss or sad about their diagnosis, talking about it in groups or one-on-one therapy sessions can help. Talk therapy can accomplish a number of goals, including providing coping strategies when they are feeling anxiety or sadness, dealing with the underlying cause of these feelings, and facing existential issues such as death and the legacy they will leave behind after they have gone. In addition to more general approaches, specific therapies have been developed to treat anxiety and depression in individuals with memory loss. Because these therapies target emotions, which have a specialized memory system all their own, they can often be effective even if some of the content of the therapy sessions is forgotten. Having said that, it may be beneficial for your loved one to give you permission to speak with their therapist so that you can reinforce the coping strategies that they recommend. Lastly, we will discuss medications to treat mood in *Step 3*.

AEROBIC EXERCISE, MEDITATION, AND RELAXATION THERAPY CAN HELP

Is your loved one feeling sad or anxious about their memory loss but is not interested in taking medications or talking with anyone about it? Three things that they can do to help improve their mood on their own (perhaps with a little help from you) are aerobic exercise, meditation, and relaxation therapy. Each has been proven to improve mood and lessen anxiety in older adults. Exercise has the strongest evidence showing its effectiveness, but there are also studies supporting the use of mindfulness training (meditation being one example) and relaxation therapy. You can find more information about exercise in this section, and meditation and relaxation therapy in *Step 4*, as well as at the end of this book in *Further Resources*.

Exercise improves depression and anxiety—and may reduce agitation and aggression

Exercise improves mood in several ways. Exercise increases levels of serotonin and norepinephrine—important brain chemicals for emotional regulation—and teaches our bodies how to deal more effectively with physical and psychological stress. Exercise can help people who are isolated socialize more. Exercise can give our loved one a sense of accomplishment. It may also improve their appearance and make them feel better about their physical attractiveness. All of these things can help reduce depression and anxiety. One study showed that over 11 years, non-exercisers were 44% more likely to become depressed compared to those who exercised 1 to 2 hours a week. In fact, exercise has been found to be as effective as medication in treating depression and anxiety in all kinds of people. Lastly, likely from a combination of changes in brain chemicals plus just becoming tired out, aerobic exercise may reduce agitation and aggression and improve sleep in individuals with dementia.

Check with their doctor prior to starting a new exercise program and if they are having any new or concerning symptoms when exercising

Regarding exercise, there are two important issues.

1. Check with your loved one's doctor before they start a brand-new exercise program, especially if they have heart disease or a family history of heart disease, are a current or former smoker, are overweight, or have any of the following conditions: high cholesterol,

high blood pressure, diabetes or prediabetes (high blood sugar levels), asthma or other lung disease, arthritis, or kidney disease.

2. If your loved one experiences any of the following warning signs when exercising, they need to seek immediate medical attention by calling their doctor or dialing 911 (in most regions of the United States): pain or discomfort in their chest, neck, jaw, arms, or legs; dizziness or fainting; shortness of breath; ankle swelling; rapid heartbeat; leg pain; or any other symptoms you or they are concerned about. If they would not be able to remember that they had such symptoms or to call their doctor or 911 for help, then they will need to be supervised when exercising.

An ideal exercise program includes at least 30 minutes daily of aerobic exercise plus additional exercise for strength, balance, and flexibility each week

The Centers for Disease Control and Prevention, the American Congress of Sports Medicine, and the National Institutes of Health all agree that the minimum recommended amount of exercise is 30 minutes of moderate aerobic activity on most—and optimally all—days of the week. Aerobic exercises are activities that get your loved one breathing harder and get their heart beating faster. An example of moderate aerobic activity is taking a brisk walk. Is a 30-minute walk too long? Shorter bursts of exercise, just 10 minutes at a time, can also improve overall health if these bursts add up to at least 30 minutes each day.

Although the majority of research has focused on the benefits of aerobic exercise, there is evidence that resistance training contributes to a modest improvement in many vascular risk factors. For this reason, we also recommend two sessions a week to improve balance and muscle function, such as yoga, tai chi, and isometric weight training.

For the vast majority of adults, there is some form of physical activity that can be performed safely even in the presence of seemingly significant obstacles. For example, individuals with leg amputations can engage—and excel—in highly demanding sports. Even those individuals unable to stand can perform a *sitting* exercise program that provides a very vigorous workout. There is an exercise program out there for just about everyone. In addition to walking, your loved one can try a stationary bicycle or one of the other machines available at fitness clubs and YMCAs, such as a treadmill, elliptical, or stair climber. Walking in a shallow pool and swimming are also great ways to get aerobic exercise—and are some of the best forms of exercise if your loved one is having any pain in their joints, such as arthritis. If they are already participating in sports such as tennis, golf, hockey, or skiing, keep those activities going! Lastly, note that there has been no identified point of diminishing returns when it comes to exercise and brain health—the more the better. As long as their heart, joints, muscles, and other parts of their body can do more exercise than 30 minutes a day, consider encouraging them to do more.

The physical benefits of exercise

Exercise helps us maintain a healthy weight, control blood sugar levels, lower "bad" and raise "good" cholesterol levels, strengthen the heart, and keep blood pressure at a desirable level—all factors that reduce the risk of heart disease and stroke. Exercise helps keep our lungs healthy, reducing fatigue and shortness of breath in those with chronic lung problems. When the heart and lungs are healthy and working well, everyone has more energy to tackle everyday tasks—including those related to caregiving. Exercise helps to maintain the mobility and function of bones and joints, reducing susceptibility to osteoporosis and arthritis. In those who have arthritis, exercise helps to reduce joint pain and stiffness. If all that isn't enough, studies have shown that those who exercise regularly are less likely to catch a cold and recover faster from a cold when they do get one.

Exercise can strengthen your own memory

Lastly, as you observe the failing memory of your loved one, you may begin to worry about your own cognitive health. In addition to all the benefits of exercise we have just listed, exercise can help keep your memory sharp by actually growing new brain cells! We discuss this topic in more detail in our book *Seven Steps to Managing Your Memory*, but here we will simply say that exercise has been shown to improve memory and thinking due to the release of chemicals in the brain that promote learning and help grow new neurons in the brain, particularly in the hippocampus, the memory center of the brain. Those who exercise have been found to develop dementia less often and later in life compared to those who don't.

SUMMARY

It is important to address your loved one's emotional problems. Learn to recognize the signs of depression and anxiety. Help them to deal with the sadness and frustration that often come with declining abilities. Start by improving your loved one's abilities and adjust tasks to make them easier. Treat depression and anxiety with aerobic exercise, meditation, relaxation, and talk therapy.

Let's consider a few examples to illustrate what we learned in this chapter.

- *I think my wife is depressed, and she also has memory problems. How do I know if the memory problems are causing the depression or if it's the other way around?*
  - Because it can be difficult to sort out whether depression or memory is the underlying problem, it may be helpful to have your wife evaluated by a neuropsychologist, neurologist, psychiatrist, or other memory specialist.
- *My husband is crying daily, but when I ask him what's wrong he says, "Nothing. I'm not feeling sad." What's going on?*

- o If your husband is crying but he is not feeling sad, he may have *pseudobulbar affect* (also called *pathological laughing and crying*). This means the dementia has made it difficult for him to control his tears, even when nothing is upsetting him.
- *My wife is depressed and anxious, but she refuses to take medications or talk to anyone about her feelings. Is there anything else we can do?*
  - o Yes! Aerobic exercise, meditation, and relaxation therapy can each help to improve mood and reduce anxiety.

9

How to manage behavioral problems

Dementia can cause a multitude of behavioral problems such as apathy, irritability, agitation, aggression, and "sundowning." In this chapter we will explain how dysfunction of the brain can lead to all of these behaviors, in addition to willfulness, jealousy, paranoia, and a change in eating habits. We actually began our management of these problems in *Chapter 4* with the *ABCs of Behavior Change*, the *4Rs*, and the *Three Time Principles*; please review these basic approaches if you haven't already. In this chapter we will build on these general methods to learn how to manage specific behavioral problems. (Note: If you're seeking help for a particular issue and you don't see it in this chapter, please review the other chapters in *Step 2* or use the index to find what you are looking for.)

MAKE SURE THEY ARE SAFE TO DRIVE— OR STOP THEM FROM DRIVING!

Most individuals with dementia should not drive. There are, however, studies that suggest individuals with very mild dementia may still be able to drive safely—at least as safely as 16- to 19-year-old drivers can. If your loved one is beyond the very mild stage and is into the mild, moderate, or severe stage of dementia, however, they should stop driving. Even if they are in the very mild stage, it is important to revisit the issue of driving at least monthly to make sure that they continue to be a safe driver. (How do you know what stage of dementia your loved one is in? See *Chapter 1* for the stages of dementia.)

There are two basic difficulties that your loved one can have while driving. The first is getting lost. Although inconvenient, it isn't the worst thing that could happen. If they get lost, they can always pull over and ask for directions, click on an app in their smartphone, use a GPS device, grab a paper map from the glove compartment, or call someone for directions. If needed, you (or a friend) can always drive to wherever they are and they can follow you home. The second difficulty is that they may not be a safe driver. Whether the problem is driving too fast or too slow, not seeing or stopping for pedestrians or red lights, or driving on the wrong side of the road, if someone isn't a safe driver, they should not drive.

There are two ways to determine whether your loved one is a safe driver. The first is that you, another family member, or a friend can sit in the passenger seat each month while they drive along whatever route they typically drive. Make it fun—go out for dinner or a cup of coffee. Studies suggest that adult children make the best observers of their parents' driving. The second way is to have them participate in a formal driving evaluation. Some states offer these evaluations through the Department of Motor Vehicles. In addition, rehabilitation hospitals offer driving programs that can evaluate your loved one's driving and sometimes help them to drive better. Although these formal evaluations may cost a few hundred dollars, they are well worth it—less expensive than a single accident.

What happens if there is no question in your mind that your loved one shouldn't be driving but they strongly disagree with you? The first thing we recommend is for them to have a formal driving evaluation, if they haven't already. This way it is not your opinion against theirs, but an objective test of their driving abilities. If they have had this evaluation and they have been deemed unsafe to drive, or if they refuse an evaluation, there are a number of things that you can do.

For many people who refuse to stop driving, the issue is not so much the actual driving as it is the loss of independence to go where they want to, when they want to. Find alternative methods for them through a combination of public transportation, family, friends, taxis, mobile app-based car rides, and other solutions. When you add up the costs of gas, car maintenance, and insurance, many families find that it is actually less expensive to help their loved one travel without their own car. Some communities have programs where high school students or healthy seniors provide rides for those seniors who can no longer drive.

Some individuals simply refuse to give up driving, regardless of your pleas, failed driving tests, and your ability to provide them with alternative transportation. Although ordinarily we do not condone deception, because of the enormous safety issue for your loved one and the public, we do believe that sometimes a few "little white lies" are better than an accident where someone could get hurt. For example, you might tell your loved one that your daughter needs to borrow the car for a few days and will return it "soon." Or, you've looked, but you simply cannot find the car keys. Perhaps the car is in the shop getting repaired. (And if you are mechanically inclined, you might simply disconnect the battery cable or remove the spark plugs.)

Lastly, in the *Further Resources* section at the end of this book we've listed some helpful publications related to driving safety and cognitive decline that can be downloaded for free from the internet. These publications include information to help increase understanding of how dementia might influence driving safety, assist in planning for potential changes in driving status, and support you if your loved one needs to stop driving now or in the future.

CONQUER APATHY WITH ROUTINES

OK, Martin thinks, *no more just sitting around the house for either one of us. We're going to get onto a schedule, get out of the house, and do things!*

Martin writes down the following daily schedule:

8:00 AM Get up, use the toilet, and brush teeth
8:20 AM Shower and get dressed
9:00 AM Prepare and eat breakfast
9:50 AM Get ready and drive to the senior center
10:00 AM Arrive at senior center
11:50 AM Depart senior center and drive to lunch
Noon Lunch at restaurant
1:00 PM Leave restaurant to do errands
2:00 PM Finish errands and head for home
5:30 PM Prepare and eat dinner
7:00 PM Read or watch TV
8:00 PM Get ready for bed
9:00 PM Go to sleep

One of the most common complaints we hear from family members is that their loved one doesn't do anything all day; instead, they just sit around the house watching television. We also often hear that they are less likely to initiate a conversation or be engaged in discussions with friends and family. Sometimes these changes are related to declining abilities if they can no longer perform the activities that they used to enjoy. They may also have difficulty finding words or understanding a complicated conversation. However, these problems may also reflect apathy—a general loss of interest, enthusiasm, or concern. Apathy can occur when dementia damages the front part of the brain or some of its connections

One of the best ways to conquer apathy is with daily routines. For example, make sure that your loved one gets up at a normal time and doesn't spend hours in bed during the day. Make sitting down for breakfast part of their routine. Exactly what the activities are is not important; what is important is that your loved one is doing something during the day. If your loved one needs to be supervised, engage friends, family, volunteers, or paid individuals to help. See *Step 4* for more information on building your care team. Even a brief outing or a visit in the home several times a week is better than your loved one staying home by themselves all day every day.

IRRITABILITY, AGITATION, AGGRESSION, COMBATIVENESS, AND INAPPROPRIATE BEHAVIOR ARE COMMON IN DEMENTIA

Nina and Martin arrive at their favorite restaurant. "Table for two, please," Martin says as Nina shuffles past the hostess to a table by the window occupied by another couple. "Sorry about that," he says to the hostess, "that's our usual table."

The hostess walks to a nearby table and Martin gently guides Nina there.

"I'm hungry," Nina says after a few minutes, looking at the other couple whose food has arrived.

"I'm hungry too!" Martin says, "I'm sure our food will be here soon."

Nina starts tapping the table.

"Don't do that, honey," Martin says as he reaches his hands across the table to quiet hers.

"I'm hungry," she says again.

"I know, honey, I know," he says as he turns and tries to catch the eye of the waitress.

Faster than Martin would have thought possible, Nina stands and starts shuffling toward the exit.

Momentarily flustered, Martin rises quickly to follow Nina, who is standing in front of their usual table. The other couple are looking at her.

Nina grabs a roll out of their breadbasket, turns, and moves toward the door.

Has something ever upset you and you felt like breaking something or hitting someone? What would have happened if the part of the brain that stopped you from acting on those feelings was not working? Because the front part of the brain provides the pause between stimulus and response, when it or its connections are damaged, a person may react without thinking. Because of this damage, a person with dementia may act on their feelings without pausing to think whether the action is appropriate or not. They may steal food or other items. They may gamble excessively or engage in other risky behavior. And they may say or do sexually inappropriate things, use more profanity, or make racist or sexist comments.

DISINHIBITED BEHAVIOR CAN LEAD TO SAFETY ISSUES

Martin is driving home. The traffic slows to a crawl. Nina begins to tap on the glovebox.

"Everything's OK, honey," Martin says, glancing nervously at her.

Nina is now slapping the glovebox. They stop at another red light. He closes his eyes and lowers his head until it reaches the steering wheel. *Come on, Martin, don't get upset, you can get through this. Everything will be fine.*

Martin raises his head and sees Nina pulling on the door handle. A second pull and she has flung the door open. A moment later she is pulling herself upright, out of the car.

Martin puts the car in "park," engages the emergency brake, and opens his own car door. He tries to get out. It takes him a few seconds to realize that his seatbelt is still fastened. Nina is now shuffling forward between the rows of cars.

The light turns green and the cars begin to move. Martin releases his seatbelt, gets up, and jogs around the car. Reaching her, he tries to guide her back. Some cars are honking. Nina's shaking is worse than usual. She is unable to move.

"Let's get back to the car, honey," Martin says while he rubs her back. After a few long seconds she begins to walk back as cars drive around them.

After a few minutes in the car, Nina is enjoying the ride, apparently having forgotten about the incident.

Martin, however, cannot stop thinking about it. *What would have happened if I could not get her back in the car? Will we ever be able to go out again?*

When your loved one has behavioral problems it can be distressing, physically exhausting, and heartbreaking. Behavioral problems can also lead to safety issues. Dementia may lead individuals to act precipitously without thinking of the consequences. If they are feeling angry, they could strike out with their fists or any available item, including knives, guns, and baseball bats. If they feel like getting out of the car they may do so—despite the fact that the car is moving! This doesn't mean that you need to stop driving and stay home, but it does mean that you need to plan outings carefully.

SIDESTEP WILLFULNESS WITH SMALL STEPS

Martin is helping Nina into the car to go to the senior center. As she bends down, she suddenly looks up at Martin.

"Did you move your bowels, honey? No problem; let's get you cleaned up."

They move slowly back into the house. Martin is trying to steer Nina into the bathroom but, clearly tired, she enters the bedroom and plops down in the armchair.

"You're tired, honey? OK, you can rest for a few minutes."

Five minutes later Martin says, "OK, Nina, it's time to get up and out of these dirty clothes."

Nina doesn't move.

"Come on, Nina," he says, pulling on her arm.

She doesn't move.

Martin sits on the edge of the bed and sighs. *How am I going to get her cleaned up?* he wonders.

After a few more minutes, Martin has an idea.

"Honey, I bet your feet are uncomfortable. Why don't we take off your shoes and let your feet breathe."

Nina straightens her legs, lifting up her feet, and Martin takes off her shoes. "There, I bet that feels better, right?"

Nina nods.

"Now, how about we take off those socks?"

Nina straightens her legs again, and Martin pulls off her socks.

"Now, maybe you'd like to just stand up and stretch your legs . . ."

Soon Martin has Nina undressed and in the bathroom.

As everyone who has experience with a toddler knows, when someone is being willful—irrationally stubborn—you can debate with them all day without success. If your loved one is being willful, the more you argue with them, the more they may resist you, whether it is to eat their dinner, take their medication, get into the car, get out of the car, brush their teeth, change their clothes, or take a bath. Many individuals with dementia have both apathy and difficulty controlling their impulses. They may be completely content sitting in a chair for hours, but if you want them to do something different not only can they willfully resist but they may suddenly become violent with little warning.

Sometimes the *4Rs* will allow you to *redirect* your loved one to something else and then, as you *relax*, you can *reassure* them that everything is OK while you gently help them take one foot out of the car (or whatever they should be doing).

Another good approach to deal with willfulness is to think of the *Three Time Principles* (see *Chapter 4*) and use small steps. Instead of saying, "Come on, you need to get out of your clothes and take a bath," *take your time* and do *one thing at a time*. Start with, "You've got a little dirt on your cheek. Here's a warm washcloth with soap on it; see if you can get it off." Then *provide timely praise*—"Great! You got it!"—while you continue, "You know, your neck is dirty too, try to get the dirt off your neck . . . Oh, now your shirt is getting wet. Let's take it off," and so on. Soon your loved one is naked and in the bath. Perhaps they still don't want to get into the tub? If they are resisting taking a bath, maybe they would be willing to sit on the edge of the tub and put their feet in the water. Once they are used to the warm water, maybe they would be willing to ease their body in. Or perhaps you'll be able to wash them with a washcloth, even if they won't get into the tub. If they refuse to get into the car to go to the doctor's office, maybe they'd be willing to go for a walk, which just happens to end up in front of the car.

MANAGE AGITATION, AGGRESSION, COMBATIVENESS, AND INAPPROPRIATE/ DISINHIBITED BEHAVIOR

Martin wakes from his nap to the sound of rattling. Sitting up, he sees that Nina is trying to get out of the house. Although he forgot to turn on the alarm pad underneath the doormat, he did engage the sliding locks.

The door rattles again as she tries to open it. He gets up and goes over to her.

"Everything's OK, girl, everything's fine," he says, reassuringly. "Hey, do you want to listen to some music? Maybe do a little dancing?" he asks, trying to redirect her. Martin moves to turn on the stereo while Nina tries to open the door again.

The music calms her a bit, but she continues trying to open the door.

Martin thinks about what to do. *Well, she's not harming anything. Maybe I'll just wait until she gives up. But how am I going to deal with this problem in the future?*

I know! Martin thinks after a few minutes. *I'll make one of those "behavior logs" to discover what is triggering this behavior, and that will help me figure out how to stop her from trying to leave in the future.*

We recommend the *4Rs* and *Three Time Principles* to begin to manage agitation, aggression, combativeness, and inappropriate or disinhibited behavior. Music can also have calming effects, as described later in this chapter. However, we acknowledge that there are times when neither music nor these in-the-moment approaches will succeed in controlling behaviors. For difficult or refractory behavior, we recommend that you use the *ABCs of Behavior Change*. Create a behavior log documenting the *behavior* (stamped his feet on the floor), including its intensity (caused the china in cabinet to clink together) and duration (3 minutes). Next work on identifying the *antecedents*—what happened before (told him we needed to go to the doctor)—and the *consequences* (I canceled the appointment with the doctor). See *Chapter 4* for more information.

Because the antecedents are usually the triggers (telling him that we need to go to the doctor), you can try to avoid them in the future (just tell him that you're going for a ride in the car) and you can plan for them better (bring another person with you to help manage him when going to the doctor). Also pay attention to the consequences. If the consequence of the behavioral outburst is to let your loved one get their way every time, you are actually reinforcing that behavior—making it more likely that they will engage in it in the future. *Having said that, the safety of you and your loved one is always your first priority, and for this reason you may need to let them get their way if the outburst may lead them to harm themselves or you.*

Lastly, because these types of behaviors are both difficult and problematic, it's always beneficial to discuss them with your care team (*Step 4*) so that they can provide you with support and advice.

LOOK FOR MEDICAL PROBLEMS

Medical problems are one cause of agitation, aggression, and combativeness that deserves special mention. Sometimes the first sign that an individual with dementia has pneumonia, a bladder infection, or congestive heart failure is that their behavior gets worse. It's only the following day when they may have a fever or other signs that they are sick. One reason you may not know that they are sick is that your loved one may forget to tell you that it burned when they urinated or they aren't able to articulate that they are short of breath. Another reason is that even a mild infection can further impair the function of a brain already compromised by dementia. If even a young, otherwise healthy individual can become confused with a high fever, you can envision how even a low-grade fever could cause an individual with dementia to become confused. For these reasons, anytime your loved one quickly becomes more confused, agitated, aggressive, or combative than usual, think about whether they might have an infection or other medical problem, and consider taking them to their doctor.

STAY SAFE

As mentioned, the safety of you and your loved one should always be your first priority. There are a number of things you can do to help ensure your safety and theirs:

- *Give away guns.* Accidents with guns happen even to people whose thinking and memory are normal, and they are much more likely to happen to those with dementia. Most police stations accept firearms.

- *Give away power tools.* As with guns, accidents often occur with power tools in those with dementia. Give them away to family, friends, or neighbors.
- *Put away knives.* If your loved one might injure themselves with a knife—or might threaten you with one—use childproof locks or put them in a place where they won't be found.
- *Consider childproofing the cabinets.* Most individuals with dementia do not try to eat or drink non-food items, but if your loved one has frontotemporal dementia they might. If this is the case, you'll want to childproof your cabinets or hide any cleaning fluids and dangerous chemicals. Similarly, you may need to lock the refrigerator and food cabinets if your loved one engages in binge eating.
- *Stay safe in the car.* If your loved one has tried to get out of the car while it is moving, there are two things you can do. First, have them sit in the back of the car and put the child locks on—that's usually a switch that you can access on the car door itself when the door is open. Second, if you search "seat belt lock" on the internet you will find a variety of inexpensive items you can purchase to prevent your loved one from being able to take off their seat belt.
- *Call family, friends, or the police.* If an aggressive situation with your loved one is escalating or you are concerned that it might, don't hesitate to call family, friends, or the police (by dialing 911 in most areas of the United States).
- *Get out of the house.* Sometimes leaving the house for 5 or 15 minutes is the best thing to do if an aggressive situation is escalating. Within a few minutes your loved one may forget what the argument was about and even that they were upset.

CONTROL INTERACTIONS OUTSIDE OF THE HOUSE

Martin, Nina, and their son walk from the parking lot to the restaurant.

We used to love this place, Martin thinks, *but Nina behaved so inappropriately last time—stealing that other couple's bread roll—I'm not sure they'll welcome us back.*

"Party of three at 5 o'clock for a purple table," their son says to
the hostess.

"Right this way," the hostess says.

After they are comfortably seated at a table in the corner of the
room, Martin asks his son, "What's all this about a 'purple table'
reservation?"

"Purple tables are specific tables at certain times that some restaurants reserve for parties with individuals who might have a
bit of difficulty eating at a normal restaurant. The seatings are
at less crowded times, at tables that are away from noise and
bustle, and they know that you may have trouble waiting," he
says as the waitress walks up.

"That's terrific," Martin says. Tears begin to form at the corner of
his eyes as he thinks, *I thought Nina and I would never be able to
eat at our favorite restaurant again.*

Managing behavior inside your home is hard enough, and it
can be much more difficult on the outside. The keys to successful outings are to plan them ahead of time, start small (don't
be too ambitious), consider the time of day in regards to when
your loved one is likely to be tired or have problem behavior,
and be flexible and willing to change plans if your original idea
isn't working. If you try an outing and it doesn't go well, don't
give up—use the experience to help guide the next one. See
Step 5 for detailed information about how to plan successful
outings.

PLAN AROUND SUNDOWNING

Martin notices two patterns in the behavior log he made, documenting all the times Nina tried to leave the house. The first
is that it might happen in the morning—but only when she had
poor sleep the night before. The second is that it happens most
days between 4 and 5 o'clock in the afternoon.

Now I know what I need to do, Martin thinks. *I need to make sure she gets good sleep each night. And I need to keep her calm in the late afternoon.*

Over the next week, Martin explores different activities inside the house to redirect her away the door in the afternoon and keep her calm, but nothing seems to work.

When was the last time things went well in the late afternoon? Martin asks himself. *I know! It was when we went out to dinner. I wonder . . . was it the dinner? Or just the car ride? Nina always enjoyed riding in the car . . .*

As the afternoon wanes and he can see Nina beginning to get agitated, he's ready. As she walks to the door, before she even tries to get out he says, "Would you like to go out?" She nods her head. "Me too—let's go for a ride."

Martin buckles her in with the seat belt lock and they are off. He drives around for 20 minutes and then heads for home. A bit tired, Nina doesn't protest when Martin brings her back into the house and then into the kitchen, keeping him company while he prepares dinner.

Martin smiles to himself as he writes down what happened today in his behavior log, tracking the progress they are making.

Although no one is quite sure why thinking, memory, and behavior worsen at the end of the day (often referred to as "sundowning"), there is general agreement that it does in most individuals with dementia. Theories as to why this confusion occurs include that they are getting tired; their vision is impaired by the diminishing light, causing disorientation; or it is related to their circadian rhythm.

The best piece of advice that we can give is to prepare for this time of day and try to avoid stressful situations at this time. You wouldn't want to schedule a social event for yourself right after you ran a marathon or spent a whole day traveling, because you know you would be tired and not at your best. It's the same thing with your loved one at this time of day—they're just not going to be at their best.

Perhaps you have acknowledged this truth and you're not trying anything ambitious; you're just trying to get through the evening at home without any crises. Use the methods you learned in *Chapter 4*. Start with the *4Rs*, and work to *relax* while you *reassure* your loved one, *reconsider* things from their perspective, and *redirect* them to activities that don't upset them. Use the *Three Time Principles* and *take your time* when you communicate *one thing at a time*, and *offer timely praise* whenever they do something well. Lastly, if things are still going poorly, use the *ABCs of Behavior Change* to create a behavior log to discover the *antecedents* that may trigger the *behaviors* and the *consequences* that may reinforce them.

CHANGES IN DIET: SWEETS, BINGE EATING, AND CONSUMING UNUSUAL ITEMS

Having lost the restraints on their impulses, many individuals with dementia will eat whatever sweets they can find, such as an entire box of cookies or container of ice cream. Why does this happen? Think for a minute what you might eat if you could consume any quantity of anything you wanted at any time without consequences such as feeling full, becoming sick, or gaining weight. Can't decide between two entrées in a restaurant? Order both! Tempted by that hot fudge sundae? Go ahead! Was it so good you'd like another? Go for it!

Although this might not seem like such a terrible problem, some individuals with dementia will eat almost any food that is not locked up; one such individual with frontotemporal dementia we cared for ate a jar of mayonnaise, a box of cake mix, and an uncooked steak. In these cases, we recommend monitoring the food that is being eaten during the day and locking up kitchen cabinets and the refrigerator at night. Consider removing sweets and keeping fruits, vegetables, and other healthy snacks in the house instead.

DON'T ARGUE WITH JEALOUSY AND PARANOIA

Martin leaves the hall bathroom and returns to the living room.

"Where have you been?" Nina asks. "You've been out playing pool again, haven't you?"

"Nina, I've just been in the bathroom. You just saw me leave here 5 min—"

"Don't lie to me!" she interrupts, staring into his eyes. "You've been seeing other women!"

He sighs and thinks, *Here we go again. Don't argue with her, Martin. Relax. Use the 4Rs.*

"You," he says reassuringly, trying to smile, "have always been the only woman for me."

Nina is still looking at him suspiciously.

"Now, what about a little dancing?" he says as he takes her hands and begins to hum a tune.

Nina sways a bit to his motion, and then stops again.

"Well, that's a start!" he says. "And let's put some music on to get this dancing going."

Any of us can feel jealous or paranoid from time to time. You see two people whispering together and glancing your way and you wonder if they're talking about you. Your spouse is making jokes or laughing a bit too loudly with that attractive person and you wonder if they are flirting. The emotions of jealousy and paranoia are involuntary but are usually rapidly and appropriately suppressed by the reasoning, front part of your brain, which perform a quick reality test and concludes that the two people whispering and glancing your way are more likely just looking in your direction rather than at you, and your spouse is not flirting or—even if they are—it's perfectly harmless and nothing to get upset about.

If your loved one is acting jealous or paranoid, your first impulse may be to reason with them, explaining why their jealousy or paranoia has no basis in reality. Sometimes this discussion is successful and the episode resolves easily. However, at other times the discussion deteriorates into an unpleasant argument. Understand that memory problems may cause jealous and paranoid thoughts to develop, and impaired reality testing may allow these thoughts to persist and grow. For these reasons, you may not be able to resolve the situation with logic.

We recommend that you use the *4Rs*. *Relax*, and remember that the dementia is the real problem. *Reconsider* the situation from their point of view: Although you were only gone for 10 minutes you know that, because of their memory problems, it might seem like several hours to them. *Reassure* them calmly that everything is alright, and you didn't do whatever they are accusing you of. *Redirect* them to another topic of conversation or activity. If the *4Rs* are not working, use the *ABCs of Behavior Change* to figure out what is triggering and/or reinforcing the jealousy and paranoia. And don't forget to ask your care team (*Step 4*) for help as well!

USE SOOTHING AND FAMILIAR MUSIC

There is a certain magic in music that helps to calm people down and make them less depressed, anxious, irritable, and agitated. Singing to—or with—an individual with dementia during care situations has been shown to reduce problem behaviors and enhance communication. Exactly how music produces these effects is not clear, but the effects are real. Have you heard the term "elevator music"? The term arose because music in elevators helps people feel less anxious while riding in them.

There are two musical strategies you can use to help your loved one feel more at ease. The first is to play music that is inherently relaxing. Whether it is classical, jazz, pop, rock, hip-hop, or folk, most styles of music have pieces that are naturally slow and relaxing, such as classical waltzes, soothing jazz, and soft rock. You could try one of these styles with your loved one to calm them. The second strategy is to play songs that are familiar to them—perhaps their favorite artist or album. Even if this familiar music is not inherently relaxing, it may help to put them in a better mood, reducing irritability, agitation, and aggression. You can also combine these strategies: play calm, relaxing pieces from your loved one's favorite artist or composer.

How will you know if the music you're playing is helping? If it isn't obvious, keep a behavior log and document how frequent, long, and intense their outbursts are with and without the music. You can try different pieces of music to see which works best. Give each piece a couple of trials, as everyone can have good and bad days.

Once you've found the type of music that works best for your loved one, make a few different playlists—an hour or two (or more) of music stored in whatever form is easiest for you, whether in your phone or computer or in a compact disc (CD) or cassette tape collection. Make one playlist with soothing music to help keep them calm and another full of happy, energetic music to use when they are apathic or their mood needs a boost. If, after a time, you get bored with those playlists, make some new ones.

Think all this sounds like a great idea but you're not sure how it would work with your vinyl records? Enlist your tech- or music-savvy friends and family to help.

CONSIDER AROMATHERAPY

Aromatherapy uses natural essential oils and extracts from plants that can be applied as a lotion or used as an air freshener that may improve physical and mental health. Some studies have shown that these oils and extracts can improve mood and sleep, reduce behavioral problems, and stimulate appetite. Popular oils include ginger to promote appetite and soothe an upset stomach, lavender and lemon balm for calming and relaxing, and peppermint or orange for simulation. Wondering if aromatherapy might work for your loved one? Although not everyone finds these scents beneficial, there is no reason not to give them a try!

PROVIDE COMFORT WITH REAL AND ROBOT PETS AND STUFFED ANIMALS

"Hi, Pop," their son says into the phone. "I'd like to stop by with a little present for Mama—something that she can hold and cuddle and will purr when she strokes it."

"Look, son," Martin replies, "I know your heart is in the right place, but I don't have time to care for a cat—I'm already spending 36 hours a day taking care of your mother."

"You'll like this cat, trust me."

Twenty minutes later their son walks in carrying a basket with a little blanket on top.

"Here you go, Mama, I've brought you a little friend," he says, taking a cat stuffed animal out of the basket.

Nina smiles as she pets and strokes the cat. To Martin's amazement, it moves and purrs. Nina, however, is not the least bit surprised or unsettled by the robotic cat.

"I knew Mama would like it because she's always loved cats. And I thought you wouldn't mind, since this one is easy to care for," he says with a wink.

Wouldn't it be wonderful if there was someone who could be with your loved one day and night—a friendly, familiar face who would provide emotional support and never be critical? Now imagine that someone would work for free as long as you simply provided them with room and board. Sound too good to be true?

Pets can provide this type of friendly companionship for many people with dementia. Studies have shown that many people—including those with dementia—feel happier, more relaxed, less lonely, and less likely to become upset when they are spending time with a pet. Other benefits for those with dementia may include reduced agitation, decreased behavioral problems, more social interaction, increased physical activity, and improved nutrition. Pets can even lower elevated blood pressure! If your loved one is already a pet lover, it may be a wonderful way for them to have some companionship. You'll just need to make sure that the pet is being fed and cared for appropriately. Although not everyone finds pets beneficial, even some individuals who have never had a pet find them be a delightful friend that they enjoy spending time with.

Do you like the idea of a pet but worry that your loved one wouldn't be able to care for one? One solution is to have the pet visit your loved one a few days each week. Or, if they are in the moderate to severe stages of dementia, a stuffed animal or robotic pet might be the perfect solution. In fact, robotic pets have been shown to provide similar benefits as real pets to individuals in the later stages of dementia—without the mess or difficulty of caring for one.

SUMMARY

Behavioral problems are among the most difficult ones you may face caring for your loved one with dementia. The good news is that there are many approaches you can use to reduce unwanted behaviors and encourage positive ones. Conquer apathy with routines. Sidestep willfulness with small steps. Use the *ABCs of Behavior Change*, *4Rs*, and *Three Time Principles* to manage agitation, aggression, combativeness, and inappropriate/disinhibited behavior. Stay safe by giving away or securing guns, power tools, and knives. Remember to call for help or leave a dangerous situation when you need to. Know how to stay safe in the car when you're driving, and stop your loved one from driving when necessary. Deal with sundowning and challenging interactions outside of the home. Manage jealousy and paranoia. Finally, consider helping your loved one to feel more comfortable with soothing and familiar music, pleasing scents, stuffed animals, and real or robotic pets.

Let's consider a few examples (some from the *Preface*) to illustrate what we learned in this chapter.

- *He wants to drive, but I don't know if it's safe.*
  ○ One good way to know if he is a safe driver is to ride as a passenger while he is driving along his typical routes. If you feel perfectly comfortable, then he is probably safe to drive. Continue to ride with him every month while he's driving.
- *I've never fooled around in my life and now, at 83 years old, my wife is accusing me of having an affair.*
  ○ Try using the *4Rs*: *Reassure* her that you're not having an affair, *reconsider* things from her point of view (she cannot remember where you've been), *redirect* her to another activity or topic, and *relax* while you remember that she still loves you.
- *I don't mind cleaning up when she doesn't make it to the bathroom, but now she's fighting me when I try to get her washed up.*
  ○ One way to deal with willfulness is with small steps. If she fights you when you tell her to take a bath, she might be willing to use a washcloth to clean her face, and then perhaps her neck, chest, and so on. If you have the water ready, by the time she is undressed she may be happy to get into the tub.
- *He's good in the morning, fine at lunch, confused in the afternoon, and a terror in the evening. What can I do about it?*

○ Look at the positive side of your knowledge. You know that he is at his best in the morning. Try to organize important family events and outings at that time. Recognize that if you do attend an afternoon activity, it's likely he won't be able to participate. Avoid evening events, and use the *4Rs*, *Three Time Principles*, and *ABCs of Behavior Change* to manage the behaviors at this time.

10

How to manage sleep problems

When you get a good night's rest, you're better able to tackle the most challenging dementia issues. On the other hand, when your sleep is poor, even small difficulties can cause you to feel frustrated and irritable. And if that's true for you with a healthy brain, think about how important sleep is for your loved one with dementia. Poor sleep can cause many problems in those with dementia—not to mention often disrupting your own sleep! In this chapter we will learn about common sleep problems that occur in dementia and how to manage them.

START WITH A SLEEP LOG

"You seem tired, Pop. Is Mama still waking up in the middle of the night?"

"Yes," Martin says. "She used to be up for about an hour, but these days, when she gets up, she's up for 2 to 3 hours—and she might get up twice in one night."

"Have you tried keeping track of her sleep with one of those logs you were using?"

"A behavior log? But sleep isn't really a behavior."

"Does that matter? Call it a sleep log."

. . .

"So, Pop, how was Mama's sleep last week?"

131

"Well, on Monday I woke her up at 8. She had one cup of coffee with breakfast at 9:30. We walked around the block after lunch at 12:45. She took a nap from 3 to 4. We got into bed at 8:30. Fell asleep at 9. Then she was up from 11 to 1, and again from 3 to 5. That morning, Tuesday, she got up at 8—"

"Hold on, Pop. Let's calculate how much sleep she's actually getting. So, she napped from 3 to 4, that's 1 hour; slept from 9 to 11, that's 2 hours; from 1 to 3, 2 more hours; and 5 to 8 AM, 3 more. So, that totals 8 hours."

"Okay. So what does all this information mean?" Martin asks.

"It means that Mama is in bed too many hours! You've got her going to bed at 9 PM and getting up at 8 AM plus napping for at least an hour each day. You're expecting her to sleep 12 hours a day when her body only wants to sleep 8. *That's* why she's awake for 4 hours every night!"

Martin slaps his forehead. "I'm glad I raised such a smart son. I guess I've got to change our daily schedule. Let's see . . . if she goes to sleep at 11 and gets up at 6, plus the 1-hour nap, that should be a total of 8 hours of sleep a day. I'll give that a try."

If your loved one has trouble falling asleep at night, is waking up too early, or is up for a prolonged period of time in the middle of the night, the first thing to do is to keep a sleep log. For at least a week, write down the times that they are getting into bed, falling asleep, waking up in the middle of the night (and going back to sleep), waking in the morning, getting out of bed in the morning, and napping during the day. Write down other things that can affect sleep, such as activities they did that day, exercise performed, caffeinated beverages consumed, and the timing of each. Using your sleep log, calculate how much sleep (including naps) they are getting in each 24-hour period, and determine, on average, how much sleep they are getting each day. Also calculate the average time they are spending in bed when they are not sleeping. Look for any effects of the other factors you recorded. You'll want to keep track in your sleep log each time you try an intervention to see if it improves their sleep.

With your loved one's sleep log in hand, look at their habits and sleep cycle and see what patterns are present. Make sure your loved one is not spending hours in bed doing wakeful activities such as eating meals or talking on the phone; doing so sends the wrong signal to the body about what the bed is for. It is best to use the bed only for sleeping and sexual activity, although many people do just fine if they spend a short amount of time reading or watching television in bed preparing for sleep.

Help your loved one keep to a good sleep cycle. It is best to go to sleep and wake up at the same time each day. Remember, most older adults need the same amount of sleep as when they were younger—or perhaps 30 minutes less. This means that most older adults sleep between 7 and 8 hours each day (including naps). In our experience, the most common problem that older adults have with sleeping is that they try to sleep too much. Going to sleep at 10 PM and getting up at 8 AM may sound fine, but it isn't—that's trying to sleep 10 hours a day, which is too much for almost anyone!

Naps are fine, but they should be short and they count toward the total hours of sleep each day. Brief, 20- to 30-minute naps are best. Naps should never be longer than an hour.

What about the situation where your loved one is sleeping through the night but they actually do sleep 10 or even 12 hours each night? As long as they are waking up feeling refreshed in the morning and are able to stay awake during the day (perhaps with a short afternoon nap), there is nothing wrong with that.

IMPROVE SLEEP HABITS FOR MORE RESTFUL NIGHTS

So, how can you actually go about improving your loved one's sleep habits?

First, as we just discussed, eliminate any wakeful activities done in bed.

Second, help them get into a good sleep cycle. Determine how many hours of sleep they likely need each day by using their routine when they were younger as a guide. If you're not sure, use their average sleep from your sleep log. You can also just try 7.5 or 8 hours a day, including naps. If they are already napping each day between 15 and 60 minutes, keep the nap. Try to match their nighttime schedule with that of others in the household and/or with their outside activities.

As an example, let's assume your loved one previously slept 8 hours each day when they were working. If they are picked up 3 days a week at 8 AM to go to a day program, and it takes you an hour and a half to get them ready in the morning, wake them up at 6:30 AM. If they nap for 30 minutes in the afternoon, they should sleep another 7.5 hours at night, which means they should go to bed at 11 PM. Most importantly, make sure that they are woken up at 6:30 every morning—*not* just the mornings that they go to the day program. A consistent schedule for going to bed and waking up is important in maintaining good sleep patterns and sleep health.

If their sleep cycle is very disrupted, try to shift them toward the desired cycle about 1 hour each day. So, if ideally they would go to sleep at 11 PM and wake at 6:30 AM but they are currently going to sleep at 7 AM and waking up at 3 PM, wake them up 1 hour earlier each day. It will also help for them to be out in the sunlight in the middle of the day, so that at night their body will produce melatonin, a hormone the body produces to make one sleep.

Lastly, we will discuss sleeping medications in *Step 3*. But here's the preview: We don't recommend any sleeping pills except for melatonin.

MODIFY DAILY ROUTINES
TO IMPROVE SLEEP

Modifying your loved one's daily routine may improve their sleep. When you try each of these adjustments, keep track in your sleep log so you can see their effects. Remember that some adjustments will take a week or more before the beneficial effects are seen.

Caffeinated beverages keep people awake. If your loved one enjoys a cup of coffee, tea, or other caffeinated beverage in the morning, it may help to wake them up so they can start their day. However, if they have either too much of these beverages or drink them in the evening, it may keep them awake at night. The first thing to do is to have them stop drinking caffeinated beverages late in the day. For example, if they like a cup of coffee or tea after dinner, switch to decaffeinated coffee, decaffeinated tea, or herbal tea at that time. If they are having coffee in the late afternoon, perhaps make that one decaf as well. Everyone is different. Some people will need to stop after one cup of coffee in the morning. Others do fine drinking caffeinated beverages until 5 PM. Switching to decaffeinated beverages entirely is the best solution for many people. See what works best for your loved one. Note that colas and many other sodas contain caffeine, so the same rules apply. Chocolate has a caffeine-like ingredient in it, so they may want to avoid chocolate after dinner. Other suggestions related to dinner include not eating large meals close to bedtime and avoiding alcohol—drinking alcohol actually makes it difficult to stay asleep.

Help your loved one to exercise regularly during daytime hours—it will improve their sleep at night. Similarly, days filled with activities, outings, and perhaps day programs will make your loved one tired at night. Avoid stimulating activities in the evening.

Using methods to establish a quiet, peaceful mood in the evening can be helpful. We discussed in *Chapter 9* how to make a playlist of tunes to help with behavior; you can use the same methods to make a soothing, relaxing playlist for the evening. When it is time to go to bed, keep the bedroom at a cool, comfortable temperature, not hot or cold.

SLEEP DISTURBANCES MAY BE DUE TO A MEDICAL DISORDER

In addition to the issues already raised, sleep can also be disrupted by many medical disorders as well as medication side effects. If you have tried the measures we suggested and your loved one still is not sleeping well, is sleeping too much, or is excessively tired, you should speak with their doctor, as some sleep disorders are very serious if untreated. Next we will discuss some common sleep disorders.

Treat sleep apnea

If your loved one snores loudly or wakes up at night gasping for air, they may have *obstructive sleep apnea*. Discuss these symptoms with their doctor. The doctor may recommend a sleep study to diagnose the disorder. The standard treatment is to use a "continuous positive airway pressure" (CPAP) machine, which helps restore adequate oxygen to the brain during sleep. There are also CPAP variations (such as BiPAP) and mouth appliances to help keep the airway open that work for some people.

If your loved one only snores or gasps for air when they are sleeping on their back, you can begin by trying the "lumpy T-shirt approach." Take two of their old T-shirts, put one inside the other, and sew the backs together on three sides. Put a half-dozen tennis balls inside the pocket you have made, and then sew it shut. The idea is that when your loved one rolls onto their back while sleeping, it will feel uncomfortable and they will roll back on their sides or stomach. This approach discourages them from sleeping on their back—the position where the sleep apnea occurs.

Sleep disorders may cause abnormal movements

Martin sighs as he opens his eyes. *I was having a nice dream about dancing with Nina,* he thinks. "Ouch!" he says aloud as Nina, still sleeping, kicks him in the shin. He moves back a little and observes her. *It looks like you're dancing in your dreams, too,* he thinks. He falls back asleep.

CRASH! It is later that same night. Martin opens his eyes and then jumps out of bed when he sees Nina sprawled on the floor.

"Oh no," he says, laying his hands on her, comforting her as he checks for any areas of tenderness.

She seems to be OK. He helps her back into bed and she's back asleep within minutes.

As Martin lays back down, he thinks, *The doctor warned me that people who act out their dreams may fall out of bed. Now, what am I going to do about it?*

The next day, Martin finds the interlocking foam floor tiles they used when the grandchildren were little and brings them up to the bedroom. After moving the nightstand and dresser away, he lays them down all around the bed.

There! Martin thinks. *Problem solved!*

Does your loved one move around excessively while they are sleeping or falling asleep? There are three common sleep disorders that cause abnormal movements in individuals with dementia, and some people have all of them: restless leg syndrome, periodic limb movement disorders, and REM sleep behavior disorder. If they are mild and not interfering with your sleep or that of your loved one, they may not need treatment. However, there are treatments for each, so if you suspect abnormal sleep movements in your loved one and they are causing problems, make sure you discuss them with their doctor. See also *Step 3* for an over-the-counter medication that you can try.

People with *restless leg syndrome* experience unpleasant sensations in the feet or legs, such as crawling, creeping, pulling, throbbing, aching, itching, or electricity. The sensations occur mainly at night when individuals are awake but are in the process of falling asleep. They may also begin after lying or sitting during other times of the day. Movement of the legs may temporarily relieve the uncomfortable feeling.

Periodic limb movement disorder occurs when individuals are asleep. Typically, there are repetitive movements of the legs, such as bending of the big toe, ankle, knee, and hip. Sometimes the arms are involved as well. They usually occur every 5 to 90 seconds during light, non-dream sleep. They may be exacerbated by medications, including some antidepressants, antihistamines, and antipsychotics (see *Step 3*). Because these movements occur during sleep, bed partners are usually the ones to report this problem. Individuals themselves may experience disrupted sleep, causing daytime drowsiness and fatigue.

And lastly, one of the most interesting sleep disorders is when people act out their dreams while sleeping. Usually only our eyes can move while we dream—for this reason, dream sleep is often referred to as *rapid eye movement* or *REM* sleep. In *REM sleep behavior disorder*, the entire body moves during dreams. Individuals who dream they are swimming may begin doing the breaststroke in bed. If they dream they are fighting they may kick, punch, wrestle, or try to throttle their bed partner. They may also get out of bed while dreaming (with their eyes closed), trip over something, fall to the floor, and seriously injure themselves. For this reason, it is important to move hard objects like nightstands and dressers away, and you may want to put down interlocking foam floor tiles in case they fall out of bed. Old couch cushions or pillows on the floor around the bed may also be used, although some people have tripped on a cushion, so foam floor tiles may be safer. This sleep disorder is very common in dementia with Lewy bodies (*Chapter 3*) but can be seen in other dementias as well.

Sometimes, even with medications, your loved one's movements may be so severe or frequent that you just cannot get a good night's rest. In this case, it is certainly reasonable to sleep in another bed if your bedroom or home has enough space. It is difficult to be a good caregiver if you're tired all the time!

SUMMARY

Although sleep problems are common in dementia, most of these problems can be managed without medications. Start by using a sleep log. Work to improve your loved one's sleep habits and modify their daily routines to improve sleep. Be alert for disorders such as sleep apnea and abnormal sleep movements; let your loved one's doctor know if you suspect them.

Let's consider a few examples to illustrate what we learned in this chapter.

- *My father has trouble going to sleep every night. I think he just needs a sleeping pill. Do I really need to bother with a sleep log?*
  - Yes! Most sleep problems can be managed without medications, and a sleep log is the way to start. Moreover, most sleeping pills will make your loved one confused and may actually worsen agitation the next day.
- *My wife goes to bed at 10 PM, is up from 2 to 4 AM, and then sleeps till 8 AM. How do I stop her getting up in the middle of the night?*
  - The problem is likely that she is trying to sleep 10 hours a day when she only needs 8. Try having her match your sleep schedule. If you sleep from 11 PM to 7 AM, keep her up until 11 PM each night and wake her up at 7 AM each morning. There may be a few difficult nights and a bit of tiredness during the day, but if

you stick with it she should adjust and not be up for so long in the middle of the night. Note that an afternoon nap is OK, but it should be brief and it needs to count toward her 8 hours of total sleep each day.

- *My husband's snoring is so loud that it frequently wakes me up. He's tired and irritable during the day. What should I do?*
    o Start by letting his doctor know. The doctor will likely order a sleep study to determine if he has sleep apnea. While you are waiting for him to get the sleep study, see if his snoring stops if you roll him on his side or his stomach. If it does, you can try the "lumpy T-shirt approach" as described earlier in the chapter. The good news is that most cases of sleep apnea can be treated, and so there is a good chance that your husband will be able to sleep better at night and be less tired and irritable during the day.

11

How to manage problems with bodily functions

In this chapter we will learn how the brain coordinates the activity of many bodily functions, including walking, continence, movement, and even chewing and swallowing. We will discuss why these and other bodily functions may become impaired by dementia, leading to falls, incontinence, tremors, choking, and other problems. Importantly, we'll also discuss a number of things you can do to help to manage these problems and improve your loved one's day-to-day function.

IMPROVE WALKING AND REDUCE FALLS

Individuals with dementia are at increased risk for falls for many reasons. They may have strokes or symptoms of Parkinson's disease. They may forget to use their cane, walker, or other assistive device. They may have poor vision. They may have poor judgment, leading them to reach for items on top shelves when they shouldn't, wear improper shoes, walk on slippery surfaces, and venture out in dim light. They may be on medications to control behavior that often have the side effect of making them unsteady on their feet (see *Step 3*). They may be drowsy because of medications or for reasons we discuss later in the chapter. Lastly, they may have urinary urgency, causing them to move too quickly to try to avoid an accident. Here are a number of specific things to consider trying to help reduce falls, depending on the situation:

- Correct sleep disturbances that may cause drowsiness, as discussed in *Chapter 10*.
- Speak with your loved one's doctor about whether any of the medications they are taking might be causing tiredness or impaired walking and balance. We will discuss medication side effects in detail in *Step 3*.
- Treat dizziness, vertigo, and inner ear disease—without medications, when possible. Ask your loved one's doctor if they could have benign positional vertigo, which can be treated by moving one's head and body through special positions.
- Work with a physical therapist to see if a cane, walker, wheelchair, or other assistive device may be helpful. Help your loved one remember to bring their cane or walker with them when they go out.
- Individuals with very mild dementia may be able to improve their balance and reduce falls through practicing yoga and tai chi.
- Improve generalized weakness due to deconditioning by strength training under the supervision of a physical therapist.
- Ask your loved one's doctor or physical therapist about treatments for any individual muscle weakness, whether from stroke, neuropathy, or other causes. A brace can sometimes be used to compensate for specific weakness, such as a foot drop.
- Consult a physical therapist about providing some help with other symptoms of neuropathy, such as difficulty feeling one's feet on the floor and knowing what position the foot is in. Looking at one's feet while walking may be helpful.
- Make sure that medical problems that may be affecting your loved one's walking are treated, such as Parkinson's disease, low blood pressure, heart disease, hip and knee problems, and arthritis. We will discuss medications that may improve walking in *Step 3*.

- Treat eye problems that impair vision and increase visual cues on stairs as described in *Chapter 7.* Improve lighting by replacing standard lightbulbs with brighter ones (fluorescent ones, for example) and adding lamps and light fixtures where needed. Make sure stairs are well lit. Use nightlights in bathrooms and hallways.
- Advise your loved one when and where it is not safe to walk due to water, ice, mud, or uneven ground. Avoid highly polished floors that may be slippery and/or cause glare, making vision difficult.
- Make sure they wear proper footwear.
- Remove clutter from the floor.
- Move items they need out of top shelves and onto lower shelves that are easier to reach.
- Help them avoid carrying heavy or bulky items.
- Tape, tack down, or remove rugs and carpets that are loose. You may also want to remove thick rugs and carpets if your loved one has almost any type of walking difficulties, as it may be difficult for them to walk across it.
- Make sure that all stairways have good railings, and help them descend the steps carefully, avoiding staircases with uneven steps.
- Provide opportunities for your loved one to use the toilet and prompt them to do so frequently to avoid needing to rush to the bathroom.
- Mount grab bars inside and outside of tubs and showers and near toilets.
- Put nonskid mats or carpets on surfaces that may get wet.

INCONTINENCE IS COMMON IN DEMENTIA

Incontinence is common in older adults, but it is much more so in those with dementia. There are several different types of incontinence and different reasons why dementia causes or worsens incontinence, as we will describe next.

- *Stress incontinence* occurs when your loved one has a leakage of urine when they cough, sneeze, or laugh. Stress incontinence is more common in older women and results from weakening or damage to the bladder muscles that hold in the urine.

- *Overflow incontinence* occurs when the bladder does not empty completely. It is common in men with an enlarged prostate, although it can occur in women as well. The bladder muscle becomes stretched and can either leak or spasm.
- *Urge incontinence* (also called *overactive bladder*) is present when your loved one has a strong, sudden urge to urinate, needs to run to the bathroom, and doesn't always make it on time. Sometimes individuals have a milder form of this problem leading to urinary urgency or frequent trips to the bathroom without actual incontinence.
- Some individuals have a mixture of these different types of incontinence.

Reduce incontinence during the day with a toileting schedule

Most individuals with dementia who experience overflow incontinence or urge incontinence (overactive bladder) can remain continent of urine and stool for a time, typically 1 to 2 hours. Because of this basic fact, incontinence can be reduced or eliminated in most individuals simply by making sure that they try to urinate and defecate every 1 to 2 hours. However, because your loved one has dementia, they do not realize that they need to go to the bathroom so frequently. You need to help by reminding them to use the bathroom—sometimes even insisting that they do so. Persuade them to go before any car ride and when you arrive at your destination. If you find they are having accidents after 1 hour and 15 minutes, make sure that they use the toilet every hour. If they are drinking more liquids because it is a hot day, they may need to go every 30 to 60 minutes. If you find this method is working to control urinary but not bowel incontinence, you may need to be in the bathroom with them to remind them to try to move their bowels each time they try to urinate.

Reduce incontinence at night

Incontinence at night can pose special problems. One's awareness of the need to go to the bathroom is diminished during sleep. Getting up every couple of hours in the middle of the night on a schedule can be disruptive to sleep, and even when one feels the urge it can take a long time to fully wake up, get out of bed, and move to the toilet.

There are two main situations that contribute to incontinence at night. The first is that some people will drink liquids or eat fruits (which contain lots of liquid) close to their bedtime. This habit will, of course, fill up the bladder, making them need to urinate in the middle of the night. It is best to just drink small sips of water starting 2 hours before bedtime (although it is also important to drink adequate water to swallow one's pills and completely wash them down).

The second situation is that some individuals accumulate fluid in their legs during the day when they are sitting or standing. At night, when they are lying down, all the accumulated fluid in their legs returns to the rest of the body and fills up the bladder, often causing massive incontinence that requires changing of the entire bed linens. You may have heard the term *edema* used to refer to this accumulation of fluid in the legs. It is also common in individuals with Parkinson's disease, Lewy body disease, heart disease, and similar disorders.

One approach that helps with this latter problem in many people—particularly those with Parkinson's and Lewy body diseases—is to try to increase activity during the day. Every time someone moves their legs, the contraction of their leg muscles pushes the blood up from their legs into the rest of their body. Because people with Parkinson's and Lewy body diseases move their legs less than normal, an activity schedule can get their leg muscles moving and prevent fluid from pooling in their legs.

Another important approach is to give the accumulated fluid in their legs time to return to the body while your loved one is still awake. After dinner and at least an hour before sleep (preferably 2 hours before sleep), have them lie down on the couch with their feet above the level of their heart. Getting into this position generally involves them putting their feet on the arm of the couch, or propped up on several firm couch cushions. As the fluid moves from their legs to the rest of their body, they may need to urinate several times—perhaps every 30 minutes—to expel the excess water prior to going to bed.

Plan ahead to manage incontinence outside the home

After tracking Nina's incontinence for a week in an "incontinence log," Martin sees that she sometimes has a urinary accident after 2 hours. With this knowledge, he has made a new daily schedule that includes her using the bathroom every hour and a half.

A week later, Martin plans a trip with Nina to the fine arts museum. He looks through the museum website until he finds what he is looking for: *Accessible restrooms for those who require assistance are on Level 1, next to the Visitor Center.*

OK, he thinks. *That will be our first stop!*

Managing incontinence is often more difficult outside the home. You may arrive at your destination not knowing where and how far away the bathrooms are. There may or may not be family, companion, single, or handicap bathrooms near your location. The key to managing incontinence outside of the home is to plan ahead. Make sure your loved one uses the toilet before they start on their outing. Call or use the internet ahead of time to find out the locations of the bathrooms at your destination that will work for your loved one, and make sure they use it as soon as they arrive. Bring a "just in case" bag with you including a change of pants, underpants, socks, disposable wipes, disposable gloves, and a plastic bag for the soiled clothes. If they wear incontinence underwear or diapers, bring several spares along.

Pull-ups versus diapers

Regarding incontinence undergarments, there are advantages and disadvantages to the "pull-up," underwear style versus the diaper style. The underwear style may feel more normal to your loved one and they may be able to put them on by themselves with the rest of their clothes. Just like regular underwear, they can be put on standing up or, if your loved one's balance isn't good, sitting down on the side of the bed or toilet. However, it is generally still helpful to have some diaper-style undergarments with you so that if your loved one has an accident and their undergarment is soiled but nothing else is, you can tear the pull-up off, get them cleaned up, and put on the diaper without needing to remove their pants, socks, and shoes—which can sometimes be a difficult and messy affair in a small bathroom.

Pelvic floor exercises may benefit those with mild dementia

If your loved one's dementia is mild and they don't mind contracting their muscles a few times a day, they may benefit from Kegel exercises. These exercises strengthen the pelvic floor muscles, which helps to control incontinence of bladder and bowels. It can be particularly effective to reduce stress incontinence. Although not all individuals will be able to learn how to perform these exercises, they do work to reduce incontinence within a few weeks to a few months and so are worth a try. Ask your loved one's doctor or search "Kegel exercises" on the internet to learn how to do them. If your loved one is able to do them, help them to remember to practice three times a day.

Keep the bladder healthy

There are a number of things that anyone can do to help keep their bladder healthy. Limit alcohol and caffeine intake. Quit smoking. Drink 6 to 8 glasses of water daily. Avoid constipation by staying physically active and eating high-fiber foods. Keep a healthy weight. Use the toilet often—at least every 3 to 4 hours. When urinating, relax and fully empty the bladder. Women should always wipe from front to back after urinating or defecating. Urinate after sexual activity. Wear cotton underwear and loose-fitting clothes.

INCREASE THE FLAVORS AND SPICE OF FOOD

Smell is one of the first senses affected by Alzheimer's disease and dementia with Lewy bodies, two common causes of dementia. When smell is diminished by dementia, food becomes less appealing because most of what we taste is actually from our sense of smell; the tongue can only sense sweet, salty, sour, bitter, and spicy. Loss of smell is one of the reasons that those with dementia may lose their appetite and lose weight. Diminished smell is also related to poor hygiene, because unpleasant smells of urine, feces, and body odor—which would normally cue individuals to bathe or change their clothes—go undetected.

Luckily, there are some things you can do to compensate for this loss of smell. First, try increasing the amount of flavoring. Does a recipe include 1 tablespoon of orange zest? Try 2, 3, or 4 tablespoons. Another dish calls for 1 teaspoon of cinnamon? Try doubling or tripling the amount.

The second thing you can try is to increase the spiciness of foods. Because the "heat" of spices is not part of our sense of smell, your loved one will be able to taste the spiciness of curry powder, cayenne pepper, and tabasco sauce just fine. In addition to spicing up your cooking, you might also see if your loved one now enjoys more pungent, spicy foods such as Thai or Indian curries, even if they have never liked such foods in the past.

USE HEAVY SILVERWARE AND MUGS TO DAMPEN TREMORS

Tremors may make simple activities such as drinking from a cup or eating soup difficult or impossible. Although medications can be tried, as discussed in *Step 3*, they rarely eliminate the tremor entirely. Because people with tremors experience more difficulty using light objects (such as a Styrofoam cup) compared with heavy ones (such as a thick ceramic mug), we recommend that those with tremors use heavy mugs, glasses, and silverware when eating. These weighted items tend to dampen the effects of the tremor, making it easier to eat and drink. Heavy mugs and glasses can generally be easily found. To obtain weighted cutlery, search the internet for "heavy silverware for tremor." You will see that many different styles of weighted utensils are available, including some that look identical to regular silverware and others that are purely utilitarian.

IMPROVE EATING AND DRINKING

Reduce choking

Martin moves the sausages off the griddle and then pours the batter for silver dollar pancakes. While the pancakes are cooking, he mashes up two sausages. Five minutes later he brings the sausages and pancakes to the table as he sits down with Nina. "Now, one pancake at a time for you. There will be no choking while I'm around. Here is some sausage for you too," he says.

Martin watches carefully as Nina chews and swallows the small pancake and the sausage without difficulty. He smiles as he gives her a second helping of each. She then lifts a heavy mug filled with coffee, which shakes only slightly as she brings it to her lips.

Many people with dementia in the moderate to severe stages have difficulty eating and drinking. Begin by making sure your loved one has proper dental care, including dentures if needed. Dentures frequently become lost; use a system to keep track of them.

Choking is sometimes a problem with solid foods, liquids, or both. Make sure that food is cut into appropriate-size pieces; help your loved one cut it up, if needed. If your loved one cannot use utensils, consider serving "finger foods" that are usually eaten by hand. Either way, ensure they only put a few pieces of food into their mouth at a time. Encourage them to chew their food adequately prior to swallowing. If they don't chew properly, you may need to cut their food into smaller-than-usual pieces or to puree their food. If they are choking when swallowing thin liquids, such as water, thickening agents can be added to make swallowing easier. If your loved one is choking despite these measures, ask their doctor for a swallowing evaluation, which typically includes a "video swallow" (where your loved one has an X-ray when they are eating and drinking), a consultation with a speech-language pathologist, or both. An appointment with a dietitian can also help you think through how your loved one can eat healthy foods despite their difficulty eating.

Most individuals eventually need to be fed as their dementia progresses. Although this activity may not sound appealing, many families find that nourishing their loved one can be a tender, intimate experience that they either don't mind or actually enjoy.

MANAGE DIFFICULTIES PERFORMING SKILLED MOVEMENTS AND ACTIVITIES

"Almost, honey. The blouse is on backwards. I know it has a button at the top, but that's supposed to go in the back," Martin says as he helps Nina take it off.

"OK, let's try it now," he says as he lays out the blouse on the bed, face down.

Nina fingers the button, picks up the blouse, and begins to put it on backward again.

"Here, let me help with that," he says as he turns the blouse around.

All day, Martin thinks about how the button seemed to throw Nina off. As he is falling asleep that night, he has an idea. The next morning, he finds a simple dress with no buttons or fasteners. He places it face down on the bed.

Nina begins to pick up the dress.

"No, honey. Just open it up here and put your arms through."

Nina follows the instructions and puts the dress on correctly.

Over the next week, Martin lays simple dresses down on the bed and helps Nina put them on.

On Sunday, Martin just finished laying out her dress when the phone rings. He steps into the hallway and has a brief conversation.

As he walks back into the bedroom, Nina is standing there, beaming.

"Why, don't you look beautiful in your fancy dress—and you put it on yourself!" he says as he gives her a little kiss.

Whether it occurs early or later on, most individuals with dementia experience difficulty performing skilled movements at some point. Such difficulties may first become noticeable with complicated activities such as carpentry or cooking and may progress to difficulty with basic activities such as manipulating buttons, putting on clothes, cutting food, and brushing teeth. There are two general approaches when these problems arise: Reduce the difficulty of the task and practice to regain lost skills.

Reducing the difficulty of the task or activity is the best approach most of the time. Many individuals who can no longer pick out and put on clothes independently can dress themselves if their clothes are carefully laid out, in order, on their bed. Those who cannot make a sandwich or coffee may be able to unwrap a sandwich left on a plate and pour themselves a cup of coffee from a thermos. If tying shoes becomes difficult, try slip-on shoes or ones that use Velcro straps.

Occasionally a lost skill can be regained. For example, let's imagine your loved one enjoyed playing cards their whole life and, even though they can no longer play, they spend hours contentedly shuffling and dealing out cards. If they go into the hospital for a medical procedure followed by a stay in a rehabilitation facility, they may not have the opportunity to use the cards and may forget how to shuffle and deal. If you see them struggling to do these activities when they return home, you may be able to help them relearn how to shuffle and deal. Begin by guiding them, hand over hand, showing their fingers and hands how to perform the activity. If you practice with them every day, these old skills may come back to them. And even if they don't, you can feel good that you tried your best and spent time doing an activity together with your loved one. A similar approach can be used to help with relearning activities of daily living. Remember to be patient, remember that it may take several weeks or months to achieve success, and remember that there is no harm in trying even though you may not be successful. Do not blame your loved one or yourself if they cannot relearn a skill—blame the dementia, and move on.

REDUCE SCRATCHING AND PICKING

"Don't scratch, honey," Martin says as he gently puts his hand on Nina's and moves it away from her arm. He can see the new blood oozing next to the area dark with scabs.

A minute later she's scratching again.

"Let's hold hands," he says, trying to smile, as he takes her hands in his.

Nina looks up from her arms and their eyes meet. She smiles at Martin and he, in turn, feels his eyes crinkle as a genuine smile breaks over his face.

Well, he thinks, *this is one way to stop Nina from scratching, but I can't hold her hands all the time.*

The next morning Martin looks through Nina's closet until he finds what he is looking for. He lays out the long-sleeved dress on the bed and Nina slips it on correctly.

"There, don't you look nice in your dress. Let me help you with those buttons," he says, buttoning her sleeves.

Later that day, Martin can see Nina trying to push her sleeve up, but she cannot undo the buttons. She scratches through the cloth of the dress for a few minutes, but then gives up on that as well.

Martin breathes a sigh of relief as he thinks, *Another day, another problem, another solution.*

If your loved one is scratching their skin so much that it bleeds or they are picking at their scabs before the skin heals, the first thing to do is to let their doctor know. Sometimes the scratching is due to a skin infection, rash, medication side effect, or another medical problem. Once medical problems have been considered, one of the most common causes of itching in the older adult is dry skin. Try using a soap with moisturizer built into it. If that doesn't work, use lotion to keep their skin moist. Sometimes long sleeves will solve the problem—perhaps a shirt with sleeves that button or are tight-fitting to make it difficult for them to roll up their sleeves. Lastly, a medication may be needed; see *Step 3.*

SUMMARY

Although dementia can disrupt many bodily functions, there are ways you can help your loved one and yourself. Determine the cause of any falls and work proactively to prevent future ones. If their walking is impaired, work with a physical therapist to improve it. To reduce incontinence, use a toileting schedule, decrease fluid intake before bed, and plan ahead when you go on outings. Make meals more enticing by increasing the flavor and spice of food. Use heavy silverware and mugs to dampen tremors. Improve swallowing and reduce choking by altering the consistency of solid foods and liquids and consider a swallowing evaluation. Reduce the difficulties inherent in activities requiring skilled or complicated movements to the extent possible. Lessen scratching and picking by treating medical problems and dry skin; cover the arms if needed.

Let's consider a few examples to illustrate what we learned in this chapter.

- *My father has fallen four times, the last time landing on his head. How do I stop this from happening?*
  - Begin by determining the cause—or causes—of the falls. Perhaps they are from the combination of tripping on rugs, poor vision, and reaching for things on top shelves. If so, tack down or remove loose rugs, have his eyes evaluated, increase lighting and visual cues, and move items from top shelves to locations that are easier to reach.
- *At first the shuffling feet and shaking hands were just a bit embarrassing, but now he keeps falling and can't drink a cup of coffee without spilling it all over.*
  - Have him work with a physical therapist and consider a walker or other assistive device. Make sure he wears proper footwear. Remove clutter from floors. Tape, tack down, or remove rugs and carpets that are loose. Use heavy mugs to reduce spills from tremors. If these methods aren't sufficient, speak with his doctor about treatments for Parkinson's disease that can improve walking (see *Step 3*).
- *I'm afraid to leave the house with her because she wets herself three or four times each day.*
  - Start with a toileting schedule both at home and when you go out. If she has accidents between 2 and 3 hours after she has last

used the toilet, have her use the toilet every 90 minutes. Plan ahead for outings. Make sure she uses the toilet before you leave the house. Find the location of a bathroom at your destination that will work for her ahead of time, and have her use it as soon as she arrives.

Step 3

ASK ABOUT
MEDICATIONS

In *Step 1* we gained a better understanding of dementia. In *Step 2* we learned how to manage the majority of problems in dementia without medications. *Step 3* explains which medications can help us to further manage problems in dementia—and which other medications can make these problems worse. We begin this step with a review of medications whose side effects may actually worsen thinking, memory, behavior, or function, as we believe there should always be a careful look to see if any existing medications can be reduced or eliminated prior to starting a new one. We will then turn to a discussion of which medications can be helpful in managing problems in dementia.

12

Which medications can worsen thinking, memory, behavior, or function?

The development of modern medications has dramatically changed our ability to treat—and even cure—many disorders. Most medications have side effects, however, and although some of these side effects are minor and easy to deal with, others can cause major problems with thinking, memory, behavior, or function—which your loved one may already have problems with! Moreover, some side effects are readily apparent, such as nausea or a rash, whereas others are more difficult to discern. How can one tell whether an episode of confusion is due to a medication side effect or to the dementia itself? To start, you need to know which medications might be causing confusion. In this chapter we'll discuss how to detect possible side effects as we review common classes of medications that may impair thinking, memory, behavior, sleep, walking, and more.

REVIEW MEDICATIONS WITH YOUR LOVED ONE'S DOCTORS

Different medications have different side effects for different people. If you suspect that your loved one is having adverse side effects to a medication, please consult their doctor right away. Note also that side effects may not necessarily be the fault of a new medication by itself; it could be that the new medication is interacting poorly with another one. Most importantly, medications should never be lowered or stopped without consulting a physician, nurse, pharmacist, or other healthcare professional. Seizures are just one of many complications that can occur if certain medications are stopped abruptly. If questions arise about medications, begin by discussing each drug with your loved one's prescribing doctor or primary care provider. In that review you may find several medications that can be reduced or eliminated because they are either causing side effects or not helping. If, for whatever reason, you are not satisfied with this review, obtaining a consultation with a geriatrician can be helpful. Geriatricians are particularly mindful of medications—and combinations of medications—that can interfere with thinking, memory, and bodily functions in older adults. Most neurologists who specialize in dementia or memory disorders (often called cognitive behavioral neurologists) can also perform this review, as can many psychiatrists who have specialized either in older adults (geriatric psychiatrists) or in psychiatric problems related to neurological disorders (neuropsychiatrists). Depending on their training and experience, some nurses, pharmacists, and other healthcare professionals can also take the time to sit down with you and go over the medications. Lastly, please note that even if a medication is interfering with your loved one's memory, it may be important for them to continue taking it for their overall health.

TRACK THE MEDICATIONS YOUR LOVED ONE IS TAKING, INCLUDING PRESCRIPTIONS, OVER-THE-COUNTER REMEDIES, VITAMINS, HERBS, AND SUPPLEMENTS

"Dad, what happened?" Sara asks after arriving in the emergency room.

"I don't know! I was driving and the next thing I know my car is smashed into a telephone pole and I'm being put in an ambulance. The police say I fell asleep. I think I wrecked the car . . ."

"I don't care about the car! Are you alright?"

"I think so."

The doctor approaches them and says, "We reviewed his medications. In addition to those for blood pressure, cholesterol, and memory, he told us that he is taking allergy pills during the day and sleeping pills at night. Both of these can make him drowsy and confused. They can also cause or worsen memory impairment. Have you observed any of these symptoms lately?"

Sara nods her head and says, "Yes."

"But they're over the counter!" Jack exclaims. "They can't be bad for you, can they?"

"Actually," the doctor begins, "those over-the-counter medications can cause just as many problems as prescription medications, especially in someone your age."

As the primary caregiver for your loved one, make sure you know all the medications they are taking, including prescription, over-the-counter, and herbal medications, in addition to any vitamins and supplements. Herbal and over-the-counter remedies are *not* safer simply because they do not require a prescription. Make sure that you know the generic name of each prescription medication so that you understand the active ingredient, as the brand names of medications (in parentheses in the lists in this chapter) may change over time. You may be able to get a list from your loved one's doctor, pharmacy, or facility with some or all of this information. If not, it's easy to make your own chart. Create a table that includes the following headings, and write down all their medications on it:

- Name of drug
- What it is for
- Doctor who prescribed it
- Dose
- When it is taken
- Date started
- Date stopped

By keeping a running list with the date each medication is started and stopped, you'll have an easy way to correlate these medications with any symptoms you've been tracking in your behavior log (*Chapter 4*). For example, let's say you've been monitoring the confusion that occurs after breakfast in your behavior log. If the confusion resolves when a certain medication is stopped, then you have some evidence that medication was causing the problem. To be more certain, you could speak with their doctor about restarting the medication to see if the confusion returns. This "medication challenge" might be important to do if the medication is one that is otherwise working well to treat one of your loved one's other medical problems.

STOPPING MEDICATIONS VERSUS LOWERING THE DOSE

When you and your loved one's doctor identify a medication that may be impairing their thinking, memory, behavior, or function, there are two approaches that may be beneficial. One is to work with the provider to stop the medication entirely. It may be that your loved one can do without it or that another medication with fewer side effects can be substituted. Another approach is simply to lower the dose. The side effects of many medications can be dramatically reduced by lowering the dose, so this might be the right approach depending on the situation. Discuss both options with your loved one's provider.

ANTICHOLINERGIC MEDICATIONS

Acetylcholine is an important neurotransmitter, a chemical that allows different parts of the brain to communicate with one another. Medications that are anticholinergic disrupt the activity of this important brain chemical, often causing drowsiness and confusion (the most common side effects) as well as dry mouth, constipation, urinary hesitation or retention, sexual dysfunction, and visual disturbances. These medications may also cause low blood pressure on standing (often called *orthostatic hypotension*), which may, in turn, cause dizziness, falls, and fractures.

ANTIDEPRESSANTS

The first thing we wish to state clearly is that most currently prescribed antidepressants are generally safe for your loved one, with relatively few detrimental side effects. See *Chapter 13* for some of these antidepressants that are not generally harmful. The antidepressants that do cause problems are those that have prominent anticholinergic side effects, such as:

- Amitriptyline (Elavil, Endep)
- Amoxapine (Asendin)
- Clomipramine (Anafranil)
- Desipramine (Norpramin, Pertofrane)
- Doxepin (Adapin, Sinequan)
- Imipramine (Tofranil)
- Mirtazapine (Remeron)
- Nortriptyline (Pamelor, Aventyl)

- Paroxetine (Paxil)
- Protriptyline (Vivactil)
- Trazodone (Desyrel)
- Trimipramine (Surmontil)

ANTIHISTAMINES

Not all allergy medications, cold and flu remedies, nighttime pain relievers, and over-the-counter sleeping pills cause memory impairment, drowsiness, and confusion—but many do. The ones that do cause drowsiness have older antihistamines in them—so much so they are marketed as sleeping pills in addition to allergy medications! Antihistamines are very useful medications to reduce allergic reactions, including seasonal allergies, but—as you can imagine—if these medications cause drowsiness in healthy young individuals, they are highly likely to cause drowsiness and confusion in individuals with dementia. Other side effects can include memory impairment, dry mouth, urinary retention, blurred vision, constipation, and agitation. In fact, even when taken at night these side effects can often last throughout the following day.

How do you know if your loved one's allergy medication, cold and flu remedy, nighttime pain reliever, or sleeping pill contains one of these older antihistamines? Just look at the list of active ingredients on the package labeling. Antihistamines likely to cause memory impairment, drowsiness, and confusion include:

- Brompheniramine (Lodrane)
- Chlorpheniramine (Chlor-Trimeton, others)
- Diphenhydramine (Benadryl, others)
- Doxylamine (Unisom, others)
- Hydroxyzine (Vistaril, others)

What do we recommend if your loved one needs to take an antihistamine? If they have allergies, we recommend nasal sprays such as fluticasone or one of the second-generation antihistamines such as fexofenadine (Allegra), loratadine (Claritin), and desloratadine (Clarinex). For cold and flu symptoms, we recommend that you speak with their primary care provider about which over-the-counter medications would be helpful to treat their symptoms. For nighttime pain relievers, we recommend "plain" acetaminophen without any additives or other ingredients. What about sleeping pills and elixirs? Please see our discussion on that topic later in the chapter.

ANTIPSYCHOTICS

Antipsychotics are medications that have been developed to treat young adults with schizophrenia or mania. When they are working correctly, individuals with these disorders generally experience a lessening of hallucinations, delusions, and agitation. Because individuals with dementia may also experience hallucinations, delusions, and agitation, these medications are often used in those with moderate to severe dementia— despite lacking an approval from the U.S. Food and Drug Administration (FDA) for this use. The side effects of these medications in the elderly include impaired thinking and memory; sedation; parkinsonism, including stiffness and tremor; dystonias (abnormal movements or postures); falls (which may lead to fractures and head injuries); hyperglycemia (high blood sugar levels); weight gain; increased risk of seizures; increased risk of heart disease and stroke; and increased risk of death.

Antipsychotic medications are generally divided into the older, typical antipsychotics and the newer, atypical antipsychotics. The typical antipsychotics that have more side effects and thus should be avoided in older adults include:

- Chlorpromazine (Thorazine)
- Fluphenazine (Prolixin)
- Haloperidol (Haldol)
- Loxapine (Adasuve)
- Mesoridazine (Serentil)

- Molindone (Moban)
- Perphenazine (Trilafon)
- Thioridazine (Mellaril)
- Thiothixene (Navane)
- Trifluoperazine (Stelazine)

Low doses of atypical antipsychotics may be used for short periods of time in individuals with dementia and should be prescribed only with great caution by experienced clinicians, with a full understanding by all parties that any or all of the side effects listed in the first paragraph in this section may occur. We discuss the proper use of the atypical antipsychotics in *Chapter 13*. Here we wish to emphasize the very serious side effects of these medications. Here is a list of the ones that are more commonly prescribed:

- Aripiprazole (Abilify)
- Asenapine (Saphris, Sycrest)
- Brexpiprazole (Rexulti)
- Cariprazine (Reagila)
- Clozapine (Clozaril)
- Olanzapine (Zyprexa)
- Iloperidone (Fanapt)
- Lurasidone (Latuda)
- Paliperidone (Invega)
- Pimavanserin (Nuplazid)
- Quetiapine (Seroquel)
- Risperidone (Risperdal)
- Ziprasidone (Geodon)

ANXIETY MEDICATIONS: BENZODIAZEPINES

Benzodiazepines are one class of medication used to treat anxiety. In addition to causing memory loss, these medications cause drowsiness and confusion, which may lead to falls, fractures, and head injuries. Studies have found that people who use these medications for many years are more likely to develop dementia compared to those who did not. Benzodiazepines are also highly addictive.

There are some individuals with lifelong, severe anxiety disorders for whom these medications may be indicated. Otherwise, we strongly recommend that these medications be completely avoided in individuals with dementia. If they must be used for whatever reason, we would recommend the smallest dose possible for brief periods of time. Note that any reduction or stopping of these medications should always be done under the supervision of a physician or other provider; seizures may occur if they are stopped abruptly. Some commonly prescribed benzodiazepines, all of which cause memory impairment, drowsiness, and confusion, are:

- Alprazolam (Xanax)
- Chlordiazepoxide (Librium)
- Clobazam (Onfi)
- Clonazepam (Klonopin)
- Clorazepate (Tranxene)
- Diazepam (Valium)
- Estazolam (Prosom)
- Flurazepam (Dalmane, Dalmadorm)
- Lorazepam (Ativan)
- Nitrazepam (Mogadon)
- Oxazepam (Serax)
- Temazepam (Restoril)
- Triazolam (Halcion)

DIZZINESS AND VERTIGO MEDICATIONS

Feeling dizzy and, in particular, experiencing vertigo (the feeling that you or the room is spinning) can be quite disabling. Sometimes the vertigo is caused by an inner ear problem that can be cured by moving one's head through a series of positions.

Sometimes it is from an inner ear infection and one will need to spend a day or two in bed or on the couch. In this latter situation, a day or two of medication can reduce the unpleasant vertigo sensation and accompanying nausea. Similarly, if you become seasick, an anti-vertigo medication can help while you are on the boat. However, medications for vertigo should never be used for more than a few days. These medications tend to be either anticholinergic medications (see the earlier section on anticholinergic medications), antihistamines (see the earlier section on antihistamines), or benzodiazepines (see the earlier section on anxiety medications) and cause memory impairment, drowsiness, and confusion. Medications for vertigo that should not be used for more than a few days include:

- Clonazepam (Klonopin) (benzodiazepine)
- Diazepam (Valium) (benzodiazepine)
- Dimenhydrinate (Dramamine) (anticholinergic)
- Lorazepam (Ativan) (benzodiazepine)
- Meclizine (Antivert, Vertin) (anticholinergic)
- Metoclopramide (Reglan)
- Promethazine (Phenadoz, Phenergan, Promethegan) (antihistamine)
- Scopolamine (also known as hyoscine, anticholinergic)

INCONTINENCE
MEDICATIONS: ANTISPASMODICS

Incontinence is one of the most common and troublesome problems in dementia and, when frequent and protracted, often leads families to place their loved one in a facility. For this reason, we think it is not only acceptable but also important to treat incontinence—even though the medications we list here may have anticholinergic side effects (see the earlier section on anticholinergic medications). However, if your loved one is taking one of these medications yet incontinence is still a significant problem—such that they wear absorbent undergarments constantly or have very frequent accidents—the incontinence medication may be causing side effects without any beneficial effects. In that case you should speak with their doctor about stopping it.

Not sure if the incontinence medication is helping or not? Speak with their doctor about a trial off the medication and see if it makes a difference. If the incontinence becomes worse, you can always restart the medication.

Lastly, not all medications to treat incontinence have these anticholinergic side effects, but the ones that are listed here do. Speak with your loved one's doctor about whether a different class of incontinence medications without anticholinergic side effects may work for them.

Anticholinergic incontinence medications likely to cause memory impairment, drowsiness, and confusion include:

- Darifenacin (Enablex)
- Fesoterodine (Toviaz)
- Flavoxate (Urispas)
- Oxybutynin (Ditropan)
- Solifenacin (Vesicare)
- Tolterodine (Detrol)
- Trospium (Sanctura) (may have relatively fewer side effects)

MIGRAINE MEDICATIONS

Migraines are a specific type of throbbing headache associated with nausea and photophobia (aversion to light) that may be disabling for an individual for a period of hours or even days. Many of the newer medications used to treat migraines are safe for use in those with dementia. However, some migraine medications can cause memory impairment, drowsiness, confusion, and other side effects in people with dementia. If your loved one is taking a medication listed here for their migraines, discuss alternative medications with their doctor. Common migraine medications likely to cause memory impairment, drowsiness, and confusion include:

- Amitriptyline (Elavil, Endep), nortriptyline (Pamelor, Aventyl), imipramine (Tofranil), doxepin (Adapin, Sinequan), protriptyline (Vivactil), and other anticholinergic antidepressants (see the earlier section on antidepressants)
- Butalbital–acetaminophen–caffeine (Fioricet, Vanatol LQ, Vanatol S, Esgic, Capacet, and Zebutal), butalbital–aspirin–caffeine (Fiorinal), and other butalbital-containing medications
- Codeine–acetaminophen (Tylenol–Codeine #3), oxycodone–acetaminophen (Percocet), and other narcotics (see the section on narcotics later in this chapter)
- Topiramate (Topamax), divalproex sodium (valproic acid and sodium valproate) (Depakote), gabapentin (Neurontin), and other seizure medications (see the section on seizure medications later in this chapter)

MUSCLE RELAXANTS

Muscle spasms can be disabling, causing pain and stiffness. To treat muscle spasms, we always recommend starting with hydration, magnesium oxide, and electrolytes; check with your loved one's doctor to see if that would be a good remedy for them. The muscle relaxants listed here may cause memory impairment, drowsiness, and confusion in individuals with dementia. Although taking one of these medications once or twice a month may not cause difficulties, we strongly recommend against taking these medications every day. Muscle relaxants likely to cause memory impairment, drowsiness, and confusion include:

- Baclofen (Lioresal)
- Carisoprodol (Soma)
- Chlorzoxazone (Lorzone)
- Cyclobenzaprine (Flexeril)

- Metaxalone (Skelaxin) (may have relatively fewer side effects)
- Methocarbamol (Robaxin) (may have relatively fewer side effects)
- Orphenadrine (Norflex) (see the section on anticholinergic medications earlier in the chapter)
- Oxazepam (Serax) (benzodiazepine; see the section on anxiety medications earlier in the chapter)
- Tizanidine (Zanaflex)

NARCOTICS: OPIOIDS

Depending on its severity and duration, pain can be irritating, uncomfortable, or disabling. By itself, pain will impair attention, concentration, and memory. For these reasons, sometimes narcotic pain medications are needed. They should, however, only be used for brief periods of time. Studies have shown that they tend not to work for chronic pain, as individuals build up tolerance to the effects of the narcotic. Furthermore, they all cause memory impairment and confusion, along with other side effects such as constipation. They are also quite addictive. Many of these medications are better known by their brand name, so if your loved one is taking a pain medication, look at the generic name or the active ingredient to see if it contains one of the narcotics listed here. Narcotics likely to cause memory impairment, drowsiness, and confusion include:

- Alfentanil
- Buprenorphine (Belbuca, Probuphine, Buprenex)
- Codeine (in Tylenol–Codeine #3 and some cough syrups)
- Fentanyl (Actiq, Duragesic, Fentora, Abstral, Onsolis)
- Hydrocodone (Hysingla, Zohydro, in Vicodin, Lorcet, others)
- Hydromorphone (Dilaudid, Exalgo)
- Levorphanol (Levo-Dromoran)
- Meperidine (Demerol)
- Methadone (Dolophine, Methadose)
- Morphine (MS Contin, Kadian, Morphabond)
- Nalbuphine (Nalbuphine)

- Opium
- Oxycodone (OxyContin, Oxaydo in Percocet, Roxicet)
- Oxymorphone (Opana)
- Pentazocine (Talwin)
- Propoxyphene (Darvon)
- Remifentanil (Ultiva)
- Sufentanil (Dsuvia, Sufenta)
- Tapentadol (Nucynta)
- Tramadol (ConZip, Ultram)

NAUSEA, STOMACH, AND BOWEL MEDICATIONS

Whether it is nausea, vomiting, diarrhea, constipation, or abdominal pain, no one is happy if their stomach or other parts of their gastrointestinal tract are upset. Most gastrointestinal medications do not cause problems in individuals with dementia, but the ones listed here may. Sometimes, one of these listed medications may be necessary. We would, however, recommend that these medications be used as briefly as possible, as they are either anticholinergic (see the earlier section on anticholinergic medications), antihistamines (see the earlier section on antihistamines), antipsychotics (see the earlier section on antipsychotics), or benzodiazepines (see the earlier section on anxiety medications) or can otherwise cause memory impairment, drowsiness, and confusion. Nausea, stomach, and bowel medications likely to cause memory impairment, drowsiness, and confusion include:

- Chlordiazepoxide (Librium) (benzodiazepine)
- Clidinium (Librax) (anticholinergic)
- Dicyclomine (Bentyl) (anticholinergic)
- Diphenhydramine (Benadryl, others) (antihistamine)
- Glycopyrrolate (Cuvposa, Glycate, Robinul) (anticholinergic)
- Haloperidol (Haldol) (antipsychotic)

- Hyoscyamine (also known as scopolamine) (Levsin, Hyosyne, Oscimin) (anticholinergic)
- Lorazepam (Ativan) (benzodiazepine)
- Methylscopolamine (Extendryl, AlleRx, Rescon, Pamine) (anticholinergic)
- Metoclopramide (Reglan)
- Prochlorperazine (Compro) (antipsychotic)
- Propantheline (Pro-Banthine) (anticholinergic)

SEIZURE MEDICATIONS: ANTICONVULSANTS

Anticonvulsants are prescribed not only for seizures but also for nerve pain, peripheral neuropathy, headaches, mood stabilization, and agitation. Luckily, for all of these conditions—including seizures—there are many different medications that your loved one's doctor can prescribe. Here we list the anticonvulsants that are most likely to cause memory impairment, drowsiness, and confusion:

- Clobazam (Onfi) (a benzodiazepine, see the section on anxiety medications earlier in the chapter)
- Clonazepam (Klonopin) (benzodiazepine)
- Diazepam (Valium) (benzodiazepine)
- Divalproex sodium (valproic acid and sodium valproate) (Depakote) (This medication is frequently prescribed for behavioral problems and agitation despite studies showing that it does not help these problems and often makes things worse. It may also cause or exacerbate tremors. We recommend it *never* be used for individuals with dementia for behavioral problems and agitation unless they are thought to have seizures, bipolar disease, or a related disorder.)
- Gabapentin (side effects may be tolerable when used in low doses [100 to 300 mg per day])
- Lorazepam (Ativan) (benzodiazepine)
- Nitrazepam (Mogadon) (benzodiazepine)

- Phenobarbital
- Phenytoin (Dilantin)
- Pregabalin (Lyrica)
- Primidone (Mysoline)
- Sodium valproate (see "divalproex sodium" earlier in the list)
- Tiagabine (Gabitril)
- Topiramate (Trokendi, Qudexy, Topamax)
- Valproic acid (see "divalproex sodium" earlier in the list)
- Vigabatrin (Sabril)

SLEEPING MEDICATIONS

Sleeping difficulties are among the most common problems reported in individuals with dementia. Often these problems are related to trying to sleep more than 8 hours per day or other factors that can be treated without medications. See *Chapter 10* for how to treat sleep problems without medications. Listed here are medications used for sleep problems that frequently cause memory impairment and confusion—even the next day. We do not recommend regular use of any of these medications. (The only medications that we do recommend for sleep problems are melatonin and acetaminophen.) Medications used for sleep problems that are likely to cause memory impairment and confusion the next day include:

- Amitriptyline (Elavil, Endep) (see the earlier section on antidepressants)
- Clonazepam (Klonopin) (benzodiazepine, see the earlier section on anxiety medications)
- Diphenhydramine (Benadryl, in Advil PM, Tylenol PM, others) (see the earlier section on antihistamines)
- Doxepin (Adapin, Sinequan) (see the earlier section on antidepressants)
- Estazolam (Prosom) (benzodiazepine)
- Eszopiclone (Lunesta) (similar to benzodiazepines)
- Flurazepam (Dalmane, Dalmadorm) (benzodiazepine)

- Gabapentin (Neurontin) (see the earlier section on anticonvulsants)
- Lorazepam (Ativan) (benzodiazepine)
- Mirtazapine (Remeron) (see the earlier section on antidepressants)
- Quetiapine (Seroquel) (see the earlier section on antipsychotics)
- Ramelteon (Rozerem) (similar to benzodiazepines)
- Suvorexant (Belsomra) (similar to benzodiazepines)
- Temazepam (Restoril) (benzodiazepine)
- Trazodone (Desyrel) (see the earlier section on antidepressants)
- Triazolam (Halcion) (benzodiazepine)
- Zaleplon (Sonata) (similar to benzodiazepines)
- Zolpidem (Ambien, ZolpiMist) (similar to benzodiazepines)

TREMOR MEDICATIONS

Depending on the type and severity, tremors can range from merely embarrassing to outright disabling. Although the beta-blocker class of medications to treat essential tremor is generally safe, other medications used to treat tremors are anticholinergic or otherwise suppress brain function. Tremor medications likely to cause memory impairment, drowsiness, and confusion include:

- Benztropine (Cogentin) (anticholinergic)
- Hyoscyamine (Levsin, Hyosyne, Oscimin) (anticholinergic)
- Primidone (Mysoline) (see the section on seizure medications earlier in the chapter)
- Trihexyphenidyl (Artane) (anticholinergic)

HERBAL REMEDIES

For a variety of reasons, many people take herbal remedies in addition to or instead of conventional medications. There are several issues with these medicines that are not widely understood.

Herbal medications are just another type of medication with their own side effects; they are not intrinsically safer just because they are herbal. Herbal medications may interact with conventional medications, so one should always discuss their use with one's doctor. Lastly, because herbal medicines are not standardized, different brands—and even different bottles of the same brand—may contain varying amounts of the active ingredients. Common herbal medications used in individuals with dementia and their major side effects include:

- Ephedra (ma huang): insomnia, nervousness, tremor, headache, seizure, high blood pressure, heart problems, strokes, kidney stones
- Kava: sedation, confusion, abnormal movements
- Ginkgo biloba: bleeding (Note: There is no evidence that ginkgo biloba improves memory, and we do not recommend its use.)
- St. John's wort: fatigue, dizziness, confusion, dry mouth, stomach upset

CHOLESTEROL-LOWERING MEDICATIONS DO NOT CAUSE MEMORY PROBLEMS

You may notice that cholesterol-lowering drugs, so-called statins, are not on this list of medications that often cause memory impairment. Although there are conflicting claims in the medical literature, the best evidence that statins do not cause memory problems is from a study that evaluated whether these medications could actually improve memory. The carefully conducted study found that statins do not improve memory, but neither do they impair it. So, if your loved one is taking a statin medication to lower their cholesterol, there is no reason that they should not continue to do so.

ALCOHOL

Although not exactly a medication, alcohol can cause memory impairment, drowsiness, confusion, and falls, just like other substances described in this chapter. In fact, as most of us know either from our own experience or observing those around us, even a single alcoholic drink—whether it is a 12-ounce beer, a 5-ounce glass of wine, or 1 ounce of liquor in a cocktail—will impair thinking, memory, and judgment. Because we want to keep your loved one's memory as sharp as possible, we recommend that they do not drink any alcohol.

What if your loved one really enjoys having a glass of alcohol? Our first recommendation would be to try one of the many nonalcoholic beers, wines, and cocktails available. The taste and variety of these nonalcoholic drinks has improved and expanded over the last few years.

Is one alcoholic beverage per day acceptable? We do not recommend that anyone with dementia drink alcohol. However, if they have no more than one alcoholic beverage per day, they are unlikely to permanently damage their brain. But the alcohol will still cause impairment in thinking, memory, and judgment and may lead to drowsiness, confusion, and falls.

Lastly, when alcohol use is heavy for a prolonged period of time, permanent damage to the brain can occur (see "alcohol-related dementia" in the *Glossary*).

ANESTHESIA

Does general anesthesia cause long-lasting memory impairment or dementia? If your loved one needs to undergo surgery, should they have general anesthesia? Family members ask us these questions every day. Our review of the available medical literature suggests that general anesthesia, properly administered, does not cause permanent memory impairment or dementia. It may, however, cause your loved one to experience serious confusion, making a hospitalization prolonged and unpleasant. It may also bring out symptoms of memory loss and dementia that were not yet apparent in daily life. For these last two reasons, we recommend that local or spinal anesthesia be used whenever the surgeon and anesthesiologist feel it is safe to do so. If, however, your loved one might move during the surgical procedure when they need to hold still, then general anesthesia will be the safest method.

CANCER CHEMOTHERAPY AND RADIATION THERAPY

Success rates for treating cancer have continued to rise over the last 50 years, in large part due to innovative combinations of chemotherapy and radiation therapy. We have also seen cancer drugs become less toxic and less likely to cause permanent injury to organs in the body, including the brain. Similarly, radiation therapy has become safer as it has become more focused on the cancer and not the surrounding healthy tissue. Nevertheless, some types of chemotherapy and radiation therapy are associated with risks of brain damage. Make sure that you discuss all possible risks of these therapies—including risk to brain function—with your loved one's doctors.

SUMMARY

Many medications may cause memory impairment, drowsiness, and confusion. Make sure that you know and keep track of all the medications your loved one is taking, including prescription medications, over-the-counter medications, vitamins, herbs, and supplements. Review these medications with their doctor. When possible, stop or lower the dose of medications that are causing problems. There are a variety of medications that can produce impairments in thinking and memory, including anticholinergic medications; antidepressants; antihistamines; antipsychotics; anxiety medications (benzodiazepines); dizziness and vertigo medications; incontinence medications (antispasmodics); migraine medications; muscle relaxants; narcotics (opioids); nausea, stomach, and bowel medications;

seizure medications (anticonvulsants); sleeping medications; tremor medications; and herbal remedies. Consider anesthesia and cancer treatments carefully. Lastly, note that cholesterol-lowering medications do not cause memory problems.

Let's consider a few examples to illustrate what we learned in this chapter.

- *I've reviewed my father's prescriptions with his doctor, and they are all fine. However, he's also taking a lot of over-the-counter medications and herbal supplements. Is it important to review those too?*
  - Yes! Many over-the-counter medications and herbal remedies can also cause memory impairment, drowsiness, confusion, or other problems. It is important to track those medications and remedies as well and discuss them with his doctor.
- *My mother is taking many medications on this list, including an anticholinergic antidepressant, an atypical antipsychotic, a benzodiazepine, and a seizure medication as a mood stabilizer. But she's had psychiatric problems for years, and I worry that she may need all of these. What should I do?*
  - Speak with her treating psychiatrist about whether some of these medications could be replaced with ones with fewer cognitive side effects. For example, can the anticholinergic antidepressant and the benzodiazepine both be replaced with sertraline (discussed in *Chapter 13*)?
- *My wife has been taking sleeping pills for years. Is it really important for her to stop them?*
  - Studies now suggest that when sleeping pills are taken every day, they can not only interfere with memory the next day but may also increase the risk of developing dementia later in life. We do recommend that she try to lessen or eliminate her sleeping pills. Even lowering the dose or reducing how often she takes them is beneficial.

13

Which medications can improve thinking, memory, behavior, or function?

Now that we have discussed the medications that could be causing problems, we are ready to turn to the medications that may help. Depending on your loved one's difficulties, you and their doctor may want to try one of these potentially beneficial medications to see if it can improve their thinking, memory, behavior, or function. Just make sure their doctor discontinues the medication if it is not working or if it is causing bothersome side effects.

WHY TRY A NEW MEDICATION?

You may wonder how a medication could possibly help someone with dementia, since no medication can regrow lost brain cells. The answer is that some of the brain cells destroyed by the dementia were making neurotransmitters—chemicals that allow different parts of the brain to talk to each another. Most of the medications in this chapter work by helping to compensate for this loss of brain chemicals. In other words, the balance of brain chemicals is altered by the dementia, and these medications can help to restore their proper balance.

MAKE A LIST OF PROBLEMS

Martin arrives with Nina at her doctor's office with a list of all the problems she is having.

"This is a very thorough list," the doctor says as he reads it aloud:

- Becomes confused, tries to leave our house to go "home," ~6 days/week.
- Sees people who aren't there ~2 nights/week.
- Sits on the couch most of the day. Does not initiate any activities.
- Slaps the inside of the car for ~15 minutes every time we drive.
- Becomes agitated, angry, & fights me every time I ask her to do something she doesn't like, such as take a bath.
- Cries anytime something is the tiniest bit sad; ~4–5 days/week.
- Acts out her dreams, waking me up nightly & falling out of bed ~1 day/week.
- Scratches her skin till it bleeds daily, then picks at the scabs.

The doctor continues, "The good news is that there are medications we can try for all these problems. It will take a little while, as we're going to try one medication at a time."

To begin, you'll want to make a list of all the behaviors and other problems that your loved one is having and bring it to their doctor. Try to quantify the frequency, length, intensity, and other aspects of behaviors so improvements can be tracked when a medication is started. The doctor can go through the list and determine whether there are medications that can help with each problem. Note that a single medication may be able to treat more than one problem.

Lastly, it is very important that the doctor only start one medication at a time, so it will be clear whether each medication is working or not, and whether each is causing any side effects. This one-at-a-time approach may take longer to treat every problem on your list, but it will produce better results for your loved one.

START LOW, GO SLOW

A good general principle of medication use in the elderly is to start with a low dose and go up slowly. Starting medications in this way reduces the likelihood of side effects and makes it easier to determine the lowest dose that effectively treats the target symptom. Most medications work adequately with few side effects at low dosages; higher dosages often have few additional benefits but many more side effects. So, in general, we recommend that your loved one use the lowest dose that works.

TRACK THE EFFECTS
OF THE MEDICATION

Anytime a new medication is started, you'll want to track whether it is working or not. To do that, the goals for the medication should be clear and measurable. Just as we discussed using your behavioral log in *Chapter 4* to help determine whether your non-pharmacologic interventions are working, we recommend that you use a similar log to track your loved one's response to medications. One simple medication log has three columns: *Behavior, Intervention*, and *Effect*. Using a log is particularly important because most treatments will not eliminate problems, but many will decrease their frequency and/or intensity. Using your memory to track this information just isn't accurate enough. That's why keeping track is so important. Here is an example:

Behavior	Intervention	Effect
Yells, stomps feet, and bangs the counter 5 out of 7 days, for an average of 17 minutes on each of those days.	New medication introduced	Yells, stomps feet, and bangs the counter 2 out of 7 days, for an average of 6 minutes on each of those days.

THREE STRATEGIES TO IMPROVE FUNCTION AND REDUCE PROBLEM BEHAVIOR WITH MEDICATIONS

When your loved one engages in a problematic behavior, there are many ways to approach it. In *Step 2* we discussed in great detail how to manage problems without medications; we always recommend starting with these non-pharmacologic methods. When it comes to treating problems using medications, there are three main strategies that should be undertaken, in order:

1. Enhance cognition
2. Help them feel calmer
3. Suppress behaviors

First strategy: enhance cognition

We first recommend enhancing your loved one's thinking and memory as much as possible. After all, they didn't engage in the problematic behavior when they were thinking clearly! For this reason—even when the problem is related to behavior rather than memory—we generally recommend starting with the cholinesterase inhibitors and then adding memantine when appropriate.

Cholinesterase inhibitors "turn back the clock" on memory loss, behavior, and function.

Two months later, Martin and Nina return to the clinic. Martin grins as he shows the doctor Nina's medication log.

Behavior	Intervention	Effect
Becomes confused, tries to leave our house to go "home," ~6 days/week	Donepezil 5 mg for 30 days, and then 10 mg after that	Becomes confused & tries to leave our house ~1 day/week. Also appears to follow conversations better. Responds more appropriately when asked questions.
Sees people who aren't there ~2 nights/week		Sees people who aren't there ~1 night/month

Donepezil (available as a generic and as the brand name Aricept), rivastigmine (available as a generic and as the brand name Exelon), and galantamine (generic only) are called cholinesterase inhibitors because they all work by inhibiting cholinesterase, the molecule that breaks down acetylcholine. Acetylcholine is a chemical in the brain important for thinking and memory. Dementia, whether it is caused by Alzheimer's disease, Lewy body disease, or cerebrovascular disease, involves a reduction of acetylcholine. By stopping the breakdown of acetylcholine, the cholinesterase inhibitors help to bring acetylcholine levels back to normal, restoring that balance and thus improving thinking and memory. The amount of improvement observed by individuals, their families, and clinicians is roughly equivalent to turning the clock back on their dementia by 6 to 12 months. In other words, when we prescribe one of these medications for our patients, we can generally make their thinking and memory the way it was 6 months or even a year ago.

Although cholinesterase inhibitors are approved by the U.S. Food and Drug Administration (FDA) for Alzheimer's and Lewy body diseases in their dementia phases, we use them in vascular dementia as well. We also generally start them earlier, in the mild cognitive impairment stage. Our thinking is simply that if you are going to turn back the clock on memory loss by 6 to 12 months, it's best to do so when cognitive function is as good as possible.

Another important benefit of these medications is that they generally reduce the intensity and frequency of hallucinations in dementia with Lewy bodies.

These drugs are relatively well tolerated, with the major side effects related to an upset stomach, sometimes leading to loss of appetite, nausea, and loose stools (Table 13.1). Vivid dreams are another common side effect. Slowing of the heart rate is a rare but serious side effect, so if your loved one is taking one of these medications and they feel lightheaded or faint, you should let their doctor know right away or call 911 (in most parts of the United States) for emergency medical attention. If your loved one does experience a side effect from one cholinesterase inhibitor (donepezil, for example), another one (galantamine, for example) might work better for them. The rivastigmine patch has fewer stomach side effects because it isn't a pill, but the patch is somewhat cumbersome and requires you to put it on and take it off daily. New weekly patches are also being developed and may be available soon.

Most people do very well with these medications and stay on them throughout their lives. Note that these medications treat symptoms and do not alter the underlying brain disease causing the dementia. So, although cholinesterase inhibitors can turn back the clock on memory loss by about 6 to 12 months,

Table 13.1 Approved medications for the treatment of Alzheimer's disease dementia

Medication	Usual dose	Benefits	Common side effects	Mechanism	Comments
Donepezil (generic and Aricept)	5 mg once a day for 1 month, 10 mg once a day after that. Can go up to 15, 20, or 23 mg.	Improved: memory, attention, mood, behavior, hallucinations	Appetite loss, nausea, vomiting, loose stools, vivid dreams, muscle aches, runny nose, increased saliva, slowing of heart rate	Inhibits cholinesterase	Generally well tolerated. Also comes in oral dissolving tablet.
Galantamine immediate release (generic)	4 mg twice a day for 1 month, 8 mg twice a day after that. Can go up to 12 mg twice a day.	Improved: memory, attention, mood, behavior, hallucinations	Appetite loss, nausea, vomiting, loose stools, vivid dreams, muscle aches, runny nose, increased saliva, slowing of heart rate	Inhibits cholinesterase	Can be taken just in the morning to reduce vivid dreams
Galantamine extended release (generic)	8 mg once a day for 1 month, 16 mg once a day after that. Can go up to 24 mg.	Improved: memory, attention, mood, behavior, hallucinations	Appetite loss, nausea, vomiting, loose stools, vivid dreams, muscle aches, runny nose, increased saliva, slowing of heart rate	Inhibits cholinesterase	Generally well tolerated

(continued)

Table 13.1 Continued

Medication	Usual dose	Benefits	Common side effects	Mechanism	Comments
Rivastigmine capsule (generic and Exelon)	1.5 mg twice a day for 1 month, 3 mg twice a day after that. Can go up to 6 mg twice a day.	Improved: memory, attention, mood, behavior, hallucinations	Appetite loss, nausea, vomiting, loose stools, vivid dreams, muscle aches, runny nose, increased saliva, slowing of heart rate	Inhibits cholinesterase	Fewer side effects if taken with food
Rivastigmine patch (generic and Exelon)	4.6 mg per 24 hours for 1 month, 9.5 mg per 24 hours after that. Can go up to 13.3 mg per 24 hours.	Improved: memory, attention, mood, behavior, hallucinations	Rash, vivid dreams, muscle aches, runny nose, increased saliva, slowing of heart rate, appetite loss, nausea, vomiting, loose stools	Inhibits cholinesterase	Generally well tolerated; fewest stomach side effects. Remove patch slowly.
Memantine (generic)	5 mg once a day, up to 10 mg twice a day	Improved: attention, alertness, mood, behavior	Confusion, drowsiness	Inhibits glutamate and stimulates dopamine receptors	For individuals with moderate to severe dementia
Memantine extended release (Namenda XR)	7 mg once a day, up to 28 mg once a day	Improved: attention, alertness, mood, behavior	Confusion, drowsiness	Inhibits glutamate and stimulates dopamine receptors	For individuals with moderate to severe dementia

they cannot stop the clock from ticking down. That means the medication is most likely still working for your loved one even if you have noticed their thinking and memory becoming worse over time. When cholinesterase inhibitors are stopped, most people experience a decline of 6 to 12 months of function in about 2 weeks. So, if your loved one had a good initial response, we recommend that they continue taking this medication for most of their life.

Memantine can reduce apathy in those with moderate or severe dementia

Memantine (available as a generic and as the brand name Namenda) works by interacting with two chemicals in the brain. It partially inhibits the function of a chemical called glutamate and it also helps the function of a different chemical called dopamine. These chemicals are not generally affected early in the course of Alzheimer's disease or other causes of dementia, but they are later on, in the moderate and severe dementia stages. That's one reason why we don't typically prescribe this medication for people with mild memory problems.

Most people in the moderate or severe dementia stage of Alzheimer's disease, vascular dementia, or dementia with Lewy bodies do well with memantine, although it has only been approved by the FDA in the United States for Alzheimer's disease dementia. In Europe it is approved for use in vascular dementia, and in our experience it can be helpful in that disorder and in dementia with Lewy bodies as well.

Drowsiness and confusion are the most common side effects that we observe. Because many individuals with moderate to severe dementia already have periods of drowsiness and confusion, we generally want to hear the family tell us that there has been a noticeable improvement for us to continue the medication. If we don't hear that there has been a clear improvement on the memantine, we usually stop it. The last thing we want to do is to prescribe a medication that is causing drowsiness or confusion!

Second strategy: help them feel calmer

If the behavior is still a problem after enhancing cognition, we next recommend a medication to help your loved one be less bothered by whatever is upsetting them. In general, most individuals with dementia do fine until something upsets them, whether it is being asked to take a shower or being prevented from leaving the house. Several of the selective serotonin reuptake inhibitors (SSRIs) that treat anxiety as well as depression can help your loved one to be less upset. Other medications that may help in a similar manner include medications to improve sleep and those that reduce excess crying or laughing, as we will describe later in this section.

Selective serotonin reuptake inhibitors (SSRIs) help with depression, anxiety, and behavior

We prescribe SSRIs (or "Prozac-like" medications) for many of our patients because these medications treat a number of problems in individuals with dementia, including depression, anxiety, irritability, and agitation. As their name implies, these medications work by increasing the available amount of the chemical serotonin in the brain. See Table 13.2 for some of the SSRIs that work well and produce few side effects in elderly individuals with dementia. The ones that we have had the most success with are sertraline (brand name Zoloft) and escitalopram (brand name Lexapro).

These medications work by slightly reducing how worried, bothered, or disturbed your loved one is about things. For example, in the individual with mild dementia who may be depressed about having a diagnosis of Alzheimer's disease or anxious about the future, these medications may reduce their depression and anxiety by reducing their concern and worry.

Table 13.2 Frequently used medications in the management of dementia

Medication	Usual dose	Benefits	Common side effects	Mechanism	Comments
Sertraline (generic and Zoloft)	25 mg daily, increase 25 mg every 2 weeks until 75 mg. Can go up to 150 mg (rarely 200 mg).	Improved: anxiety, mood, behavior	Sexual dysfunction, nausea, diarrhea, stomach upset, insomnia, fatigue, somnolence, headache	Selective serotonin reuptake inhibitor (SSRI)	Generally well tolerated. Need to reduce dose slowly.
Escitalopram (generic and Lexapro)	5 mg daily, increase 5 mg in 2 weeks to 10 mg. Can go up to 20 mg.	Improved: anxiety, mood, behavior	Sexual dysfunction, nausea, diarrhea, stomach upset, insomnia, fatigue, somnolence, headache	Selective serotonin reuptake inhibitor (SSRI)	Generally well tolerated. Need to reduce dose slowly.
Dextromethorphan/ quinidine (Nuedexta)	1 capsule daily for 1 week, then 1 capsule twice a day	Improved: inappropriate laughing and crying	Diarrhea, dizziness, poor energy, cough, vomiting, edema, abdominal pain, flatulence	Unknown	Try stopping medication every few months to see if still needed.

(continued)

Table 13.2 Continued

Medication	Usual dose	Benefits	Common side effects	Mechanism	Comments
Melatonin (generic)	0.5, 1, 3, 6, and 10 mg. Start at 0.5 for 2 weeks, increase dose as needed every 2 weeks.	Improved: sleep cycle, insomnia, REM sleep behavior disorder (acting out dreams)	Being tired and related symptoms, including headache, irritability, daytime sleepiness, depression	Hormone produced by the body that sets the circadian rhythm	Take approximately 1 hour prior to sleep. Generally well tolerated.
Acetaminophen (generic and Tylenol)	325 mg for 2 weeks, increase to 650 or 975 mg if needed	Improved: sleep, pain, discomfort	Side effects are rare but can include bloody or black tarry stools, rash, itching, oral ulcers, bloody or cloudy urine, tiredness, weakness, bleeding or bruising.	Mild pain and fever reliever	Generally well tolerated. Overdose can produce liver failure.
Carbidopa/levodopa (Sinemet, Sinemet CR, Rytary, Duopa)	25/100-mg pill once daily, increase to 3 times a day, then increase as tolerated	Improved: walking, movement, parkinsonian tremor	Nausea, dizziness, insomnia, confusion, headache, low blood pressure, abnormal movements, hallucinations, psychosis	Delivers dopamine to the brain	Taper drug up and down slowly to reduce side effects. Do not stop abruptly from high doses.

Medication	Dosage	Benefit	Side effects	Mechanism	Notes
Risperidone (Risperdal)	0.25 mg at bedtime, up to 2 mg per day	Improved: agitation, delusions, psychosis, picking	Memory impairment, confusion, drowsiness, stroke, heart attack, death	Blocks dopamine receptors	Use only after other options have been tried. Taper down medication every few months to see if still needed.
Pimavanserin (Nuplazid)	17 mg daily, up to 34 mg per day	Improved: agitation, delusions, psychosis, hallucinations	Memory impairment, confusion, drowsiness, edema, nausea, constipation, poor walking	Blocks serotonin receptors	Use only after other options have been tried. Taper down medication every few months to see if still needed.
Atenolol (Tenormin)	25 mg daily; can increase as tolerated	Improved: essential tremor	Slow heart rate, fainting, death, low blood pressure, depression, fatigue, dizziness	Blocks beta-adrenergic receptors	Taper drug up and down slowly to reduce side effects. Do not stop abruptly from high doses.
Propranolol (Inderal) (also available as extended release [ER])	10 mg once or twice daily; 60 mg ER; can increase as tolerated	Improved: essential tremor	Slow heart rate, fainting, death, low blood pressure, depression, fatigue, dizziness	Blocks beta-adrenergic receptors	Taper drug up and down slowly to reduce side effects. Do not stop abruptly from high doses.

An individual with severe dementia who frequently becomes angry and agitated when asked to bathe may have fewer behavioral problem when taking one of these medications because they become less upset and bothered about the activity.

Although behavioral problems are generally readily apparent, it may be more difficult to know if your loved one is experiencing depression or anxiety. If you are not sure, please review *Chapter 8*, as these problems are extremely common in dementia.

Medications for crying or laughing too easily

Have you ever observed your loved one cry and, when you asked them what was wrong, they tell you "nothing," and that they don't know why they are crying? In *Chapter 8* we discussed how your loved one may cry or laugh too easily or inappropriately, and we mentioned the terms used to label it: *pseudobulbar affect* and *pathological laughing and crying.* The reason it is important to try to separate true sadness from inappropriate crying is that their treatments are different. If your loved one is crying because they are experiencing sadness and depression, we would try one of the SSRI medications we just described. But if they are crying too easily or inappropriately and not really feeling sad, we would use the combination pill dextromethorphan/quinidine (brand name Nuedexta).

You may recognize the active ingredient, "dextromethorphan," as it is a cough suppressant often found in over-the-counter cough syrups. Quinidine, the other ingredient, prevents the metabolism of dextromethorphan so it stays in the body longer.

Crying or laughing too easily isn't always enough of a problem that it is worth treating. However, it can be embarrassing for your loved one or those around them and, if it is limiting them going out to restaurants and other public places, then it is definitely worth asking their doctor about a trial of this medication.

Sleep medications

Sleep disturbances are common in older adults and even more common in those with dementia. We always recommend you start with non-pharmacologic treatment of sleep problems because these methods are effective most of the time; see *Chapter 10* for details.

If you have worked with your loved one and faithfully tried the non-pharmacologic treatments we recommend and there are still sleep problems, you may want to try one of the two medications we discuss here: melatonin and acetaminophen. Note that because both are available over the counter, you can try them on your own, but please still discuss their use with your loved one's doctor to be sure there will not be any adverse interactions with their other medications.

Melatonin

Melatonin is a hormone that our body makes normally to help regulate our sleep cycle. When we are exposed to sunlight during the day, melatonin is released in the evening, telling our body it is time to go to sleep. If your loved one is not exposed to much sunlight during the day or the light exposure they receive occurs at random times, they may benefit from taking melatonin approximately 1 hour prior to sleep.

In addition to treating insomnia, melatonin has been found to reduce the abnormal movements related to acting-out dreams in REM sleep behavior disorder, a common symptom of Lewy body disease (see *Chapters 3* and *10*).

As a hormone one's body makes naturally, melatonin is fairly safe; the main side effects are related to feeling tired—but that's the effect you want. Dosage begins at 0.5 mg and goes up to 10 mg. Note, however, that more is not always better; one study found that dosages of 0.5 and 1 mg were as effective as 10 mg. So, start with 0.5 mg for 2 weeks and see if it is producing any improvement. Make sure you use your medication or sleep log (*Chapter 10*) to measure the effects. If sleep is not improved with 0.5 mg, try 1 mg for the next 2 weeks. Still not working? You can try increasing the dose, again at 2-week intervals, to 3 mg, then 6 mg, and finally 10 mg until it is producing beneficial effects or you decide it's just not working for your loved one. If you find that melatonin is having a beneficial effect and the effect is the same at both the high and low doses that you have tried, go back to the smallest effective dose.

Acetaminophen

The other medication we recommend to help with sleep problems is *acetaminophen* (brand name Tylenol). A mild pain reliever, acetaminophen is beneficial for sleep because most of us—particularly as we get older—have a variety of chronic aches and pains. Although during the day when we are busy we can typically ignore these minor discomforts, they may keep us awake when we are lying quietly in bed at night. Acetaminophen can ease these discomforts and help your loved one go to sleep. Start with one regular-strength pill (325 mg) for 2 weeks and, if needed, increase to two pills (650 mg). You can try going up to three regular-strength pills nightly (975 mg), but always return to the lowest effective dose. Note that you want to make sure the preparation you purchase is "plain acetaminophen" without any additives. You do *not* want "Tylenol PM" or a similar "PM" formulation—these preparations contain antihistamines, which will make your loved one confused and impair their memory (see *Chapter 12*).

Third strategy: suppress behaviors

Only once we have tried non-pharmacologic methods, enhanced cognition, and helped your loved one to be more calm would we recommend trying a medication to suppress behaviors, such as an atypical neuroleptic.

Atypical neuroleptics

"Can we stop Nina from scratching?" Martin asks the doctor. "She scratches herself till it bleeds—and then she picks the scabs. For a while I was able to manage it with long sleeves, but now she's scratching other parts of her body—her hands and even her face."

"She's already taking the medications that I typically try first, including donepezil, memantine, sertraline, and dextromethorphan/quinidine," the doctor replies. "I think we should try a tiny dose of risperidone. But, before we try it, I need to go over a long list of very serious side effects so you understand both the risks and what to look out for."

Atypical neuroleptics are a type of antipsychotic medication that have been developed to treat young adults with schizophrenia or mania. They are not approved by the FDA to treat individuals with dementia. The side effects of these medications can include impaired thinking and memory; sedation; parkinsonism, including stiffness and tremor; dystonias (abnormal movements or postures); falls (which may lead to fractures and head injuries); hyperglycemia (high blood sugar levels); weight gain; increased risk of seizures; increased risk of heart disease and stroke; and increased risk of death.

For these reasons, we try to avoid prescribing these medications. When there are undesirable behaviors, we always start with non-pharmacologic treatments, as described in *Step 2*. If those measures are not enough, we begin by making sure that cholinesterase inhibitors and memantine have been tried and their doses optimized. Then we generally try one of the SSRI medications described earlier in the chapter. We may try dextromethorphan/quinidine (described earlier) as one study showed that it could be beneficial. Only after exhausting all of those other measures would we consider prescribing an atypical neuroleptic.

Nonetheless, when agitation and problematic behaviors escalate at home, these medications can help. They may be the only way to keep your loved one out of an institution. Problems that may be improved include agitation, aggression, combativeness, willfulness, paranoia, delusions, hallucinations, and picking behavior. Some of the important principles are to start with a low dose, increase the dose slowly (if the behaviors allow), and—after it has been working successfully for a time—try reducing and potentially stopping the medication every few months. Although many individuals with dementia will benefit from an atypical neuroleptic for a period of time, few will require these medications for years.

Risperidone (Risperdal) is the one we usually try first as it has a reasonable balance between efficacy and side effects (see Table 13.2). In addition, although none of these medications have been particularly beneficial in controlled studies, risperidone probably has the best evidence of any of them. Olanzapine (Zyprexa) is often used as well, although it may produce weight gain. Quetiapine (Seroquel) seems to be mainly sedating and is therefore often used at night. Pimavanserin (Nuplazid) has been shown to reduce hallucinations and psychosis in individuals with dementia with Lewy bodies. Your loved one's doctor may wish to try other atypical neuroleptics as well.

MEDICATIONS FOR MOVEMENT PROBLEMS

The last group of medications that may benefit your loved one are medications that can help with their movement by either improving their ability to get out of a chair and walk or reducing tremors or both.

Parkinson's disease medications

As we discussed in *Chapter 3*, individuals with dementia with Lewy bodies generally have symptoms of Parkinson's disease, including slow movements, shuffling walking, and a pill-rolling tremor. These individuals may show benefit from the medication carbidopa/levodopa, better known by its brand name Sinemet (see Table 13.2). When it works, walking and other movements are improved, and the tremor may be as well. At low doses this medication is generally well tolerated. At high doses there are many potential side effects, including nausea, dizziness, insomnia, confusion, headache, low blood pressure, abnormal movements, hallucinations, and psychosis.

Tremor medications

Tremors can be embarrassing when mild and disabling when severe. If tremors are a problem, the first step is to review your loved one's medications to see if any of them could be causing tremors, such as divalproex sodium (Depakote) or gabapentin (Neurontin) (*Chapter 12*). The second step is to reduce caffeine and to try using heavy mugs, glasses, and silverware when eating (*Chapter 11*). The third step is to bring your loved one to a neurologist who can help sort out what type of tremor they have.

If your loved one has the pill-rolling tremor of dementia with Lewy bodies or Parkinson's disease (or other tremors related to those disorders), carbidopa/levodopa (described earlier in this chapter) is most likely to help.

If your loved one has essential tremor, you can try a medication such as atenolol (Tenormin) or propranolol (Inderal). These beta-blocker medications are generally used for heart disease and blood-pressure control, but they can help reduce this type of tremor. Possible side effects include slow heart rate and low blood pressure that could lead to fainting or death, depression, fatigue, and dizziness. Note that these medications need to be tapered down slowly if they are stopped.

MEDICATIONS THAT DON'T WORK

You may be surprised about the medications, herbs, or supplements that are not discussed above, such as acetyl-L-carnitine, creatine, curcumin, gingko biloba, phosphatidylserine, resveratrol, and Prevagen. Unfortunately, our reading of the medical literature suggests that none of these substances provide any benefit for thinking, memory, or behavior. Our recommendation is not to waste your money on them.

CONSIDER CLINICAL TRIALS

"Doctor, I'm so grateful for all you've done for Nina over the last year. When we started working with you, I was at the end of my rope," Martin says, swallowing. "She is doing so much better, and now I can get a good night's sleep!"

"I'm glad I was able to help."

"Are there any other medications that could help her?"

"Well, she's on all the standard medications I recommend, but we're running a clinical trial of a new medicine that might reduce agitation and other behaviors even more."

The medications described in this chapter may be useful for your loved one. However, none of these medications are likely to resolve their problems completely, which is why you may want to consider participating in a clinical trial of one of the new medications being developed to improve thinking, memory, mood, or behavior beyond what is currently available. Some of the drugs in development are actually trying to slow down the progression of dementia by removing the underlying pathology causing the disease process, such as the plaques or tangles of

Alzheimer's disease. Because the current medications can only do so much, we recommend that all of our patients consider clinical trials.

Clinical trials are not for everyone. Few people want to return to the doctor's office for more visits, pencil-and-paper tests, blood draws, EKGs, and brain scans. Some people don't like the idea that they could get a placebo instead of the real medication. Other people are concerned about possible unknown side effects if they do get the real medication.

Most people, however, actually enjoy participating in clinical trials. Clinical trials are one way to actively take charge of your loved one's disease and fight it directly. The additional visits are not onerous and can provide additional time to ask questions. People who participate in clinical trials actually end up with better health care than the average person, likely due to the frequent medical monitoring. Lastly, people who participate in clinical trials enjoy knowing that even if their participation doesn't end up helping them directly, they are contributing to scientific knowledge that can bring better treatments or even a possible cure for the next generation.

SUMMARY

Dementia disrupts a number of brain chemicals, and medications may be helpful to restore the balance of these neurotransmitters. When considering a new medication, it is important to set clear, measurable goals; start with a low dose; and track the effects over time. Cholinesterase inhibitors help with memory, mood, behavioral problems, and hallucinations; memantine helps with attention, alertness, mood, and behavioral problems; SSRIs help with mood, anxiety, and behavioral problems; dextromethorphan/quinidine helps with inappropriate laughing or crying as well as behavioral problems; melatonin and acetaminophen help with sleep; atypical neuroleptics help with agitation, aggression, delusions, hallucinations, and picking; carbidopa/levodopa helps with walking, movement, and parkinsonian tremors; and beta blockers help with essential tremor. Clinical trials of new medications being developed may be available for those who are looking for better treatments for their loved one and for the next generation.

Let's consider a few examples to illustrate what we learned in this chapter.

- *My mother isn't on any of these medications. Should I start them all at once?*
  - No. It is important to start one medication at a time. That's the only way to know which medications are producing beneficial effects and which may be causing side effects.
- *My father is not on any of these medications and his behavior is out of control. Which medication should I try first?*
  - In general, we always want to improve cognition first, so we would start with a cholinesterase inhibitor, such as donepezil. If his behavior was still problematic, we would then try adding memantine. Next, we would help him relax by trying an SSRI, such as sertraline. If none of those treatments were sufficient, we would try suppressing the unwanted behaviors with an atypical neuroleptic, such as risperidone. In each case we would only continue the medication if it was clearly showing beneficial effects and few or no bothersome side effects.
- *My wife has had sleeping problems for years. Would melatonin or acetaminophen really help her?*
  - They may, but only after the non-pharmacologic approaches have been instituted, such as treating sleep hygiene and sleep cycle problems (see *Chapter 10*).

Step 4

BUILD YOUR CARE TEAM

In *Steps 1* through *3* we learned about why problems in dementia develop and some of the ways to deal with them. We also learned which medications might be beneficial for your loved one and which might be causing some of the problems. In *Step 4* we will discuss how to build your care team. We will begin with the most important member of the care team—you! We'll show you how to take care of yourself while you are caring for your loved one. You'll be able to provide better care when you are healthy and strong, physically and mentally. Next, we'll show you how to build your care team so you aren't doing all the work by yourself, including engaging family, friends, and neighbors as well as considering professional caregivers, day programs, and respite care.

14

Why and how should you care for yourself?

To be a caregiver, it often seems like you need the powers of Wonder Woman, the strength of Superman, the wisdom of Mother Teresa, and the patience of Mahatma Gandhi. In other words, you need to be a combination of a superhero and a saint. No one can do this superhuman work if their own physical or mental health is in disarray. In order to take good care of your loved one, you need to take care of yourself too! Just as Popeye needs his spinach to make him strong, you need to eat right, exercise, maintain your social connections, and take a little time for yourself to be the best caregiver you can be.

YOU ARE NOT ALONE

How much longer can I keep going like this? Sara wonders. It's been 6 months since her father, Jack, crashed his car into a tree. Jack didn't argue when she put a stop to his driving, nor did he argue about not taking the sleeping pills anymore. He did better, at least for a few months. Today, however, he is as forgetful as ever.

These days, Sara stops by her father's house every morning to make sure he gets up, has breakfast, and takes all of his pills.

And she takes him to the doctor. And the supermarket. And the bank. And everywhere else he needs to go.

Sara sighs as she rolls over and tries to go to sleep. She knows what she is now. In addition to working full time and being a single parent to her daughter, she's now a care partner to her father. She loves her father and wants to give back to him for all the years he spent raising her. But it just doesn't seem fair.

I don't even have five minutes to myself, she thinks as she rolls the other way, still searching for sleep.

You are one of more than 16 million unpaid caregivers for those with Alzheimer's disease and other dementias in the United States alone, providing more than 18 billion hours of care valued at over $230 billion. Caregivers are usually family members, although sometimes friends provide care. Two out of three caregivers are women. One in three caregivers is over the age of 65. More caregivers than ever before are part of what is known as the *sandwich generation*—those who are caring for a loved one with dementia while simultaneously caring for their own children. The number of caregivers is expected to rise as the aging population grows, barring any advances in treatment for Alzheimer's disease and other dementias. To put it simply, you do a lot and you are not alone.

BECOMING A CAREGIVER OR A CARE PARTNER

We all help our friends and our family, and they help us in return. This mutual, reciprocal relationship is an important part of life. Caregiving for a loved one with dementia is different, because we give of our self with little expectation of receiving anything in return. Perhaps we feel that our spouse or parent has supported and cared for us for many years, and now it is our time to give back and care for them. Most of the time, the term *caregiver* is the appropriate one for this new relationship, because we are the "givers of care." Sometimes, however, we are helping our loved one in the initial stages of dementia by partnering with them rather than simply providing them with care. In this instance, our loved one may still be able to do many things themselves, and we are helping them achieve as much independence as they can. For this reason, the term *care partner* may be appropriate early on, when you are working with your loved one to enable them to be as independent as possible. As the dementia progresses, your role will likely switch from care partner to caregiver.

WHATEVER IT TAKES

When caregivers are asked what they do to provide care for their loved one, they often respond, "Whatever it takes." The amount and type of help that care partners and caregivers provide changes over time as the disease progresses, from occasional assistance to full-time care. The "caregiver career" refers to the transition that takes place from the start of thinking of oneself as a care partner or caregiver to the end of that role. The transition to considering oneself a caregiver can be a slow and often difficult one, as individuals come to terms with their loved one's diagnosis of dementia and adjust to their new role. In the early stages of dementia, one may not even consider oneself to be a care partner, perhaps only providing occasional reminders or help with complex activities. At some point in the process of navigating dementia, you will (or have already) come to think of yourself as a care partner or caregiver. Even when a family decides to move their loved one out of their home and into a facility where greater care can be provided by professionals, most family caregivers still provide some level of care. Being a caregiver usually ends when the individual with dementia passes away, requiring another period of adjustment as this important role ends and families mourn the loss of their loved one.

YOU CAN'T POUR FROM AN EMPTY CUP

Caring for a loved one with dementia is full of transitions, requiring flexibility and adaptation as caregiving demands change with disease progression. Some measure of stress inevitably comes with this unstable experience. Caregivers experience high rates of emotional and physical illness and are even at risk for premature death. Caregivers can be so focused on taking good care of others that they may put themselves last. This is often true for the sandwich generation who care for aging parents and growing children. Sooner or later, they find themselves trying to pour from a cup that is rapidly emptying. In order to care for others, you must take care of yourself. To be the best caregiver you can be, you need to make time to fill your cup!

TAKE CARE OF YOUR HEALTH

To start, you need to take care of your health. Although we have discussed many of these health issues in relation to your loved one, they bear repeating here in relation to your own health and wellbeing. Note that activities that benefit your physical health also benefit your emotional health and vice versa. For example, there is now substantial evidence that cardiovascular diseases like high blood pressure and heart disease can be significantly affected by stress and other negative emotions. It is also known that poor physical health can contribute to the development of emotional problems, including anxiety and depression. The good news is that there are lifestyle behaviors that can help you maintain or improve your physical and emotional health, boosting your mood and alleviating stress, anxiety, and depression. Make time to engage in these healthy lifestyle behaviors.

EXERCISE, EXERCISE, EXERCISE

Exercise is critically important to both physical and mental health. If there was such a thing as a "magic bullet" for brain health, exercise would be it! Cardiovascular exercise, strength training, and flexibility training are the core components of a well-rounded exercise routine. Just make sure you check with your doctor prior to starting a new exercise program and if you are having any new or concerning symptoms when exercising. See *Chapter 8* for more details on the best types of exercise to improve brain health and reduce depression and anxiety.

SLEEP IS CRITICAL FOR YOUR HEALTH

Are you having trouble sleeping? Sleep problems are more common in those caring for a loved one with dementia, with the majority reporting some sleep difficulties during their time providing care. Sometimes these sleep difficulties are due to the problematic behaviors of the individual with dementia, as described in *Chapter 10*, such as nighttime wandering, agitation, or moving in bed, all of which keep the caregiver awake. At other times, the sleep disturbance is a result of the caregiver's level of stress, anxiety, or depression. And of course, as caregivers age, they have the risk of any older adult for developing a sleep disorder such as insomnia (difficulty falling asleep or staying asleep) or sleep apnea (when breathing repeatedly starts and stops during the night).

Getting restful, restorative sleep is critical to maintaining your physical and mental health. Anyone who has experienced a sleepless night knows how difficult it can be to make it through the next day. Poor sleep saps the energy you need to provide care for yourself and others, lowers your ability to manage stress, and leaves you more susceptible to becoming irritated with your loved one—which can then worsen their difficult behaviors. Chronic sleep disturbances and sleep disorders are associated with depression, anxiety, impairments of the immune system, and poor physical health, placing you at increased risk of infection, high blood pressure, diabetes, heart disease, stroke, and mood disorders. In fact, even one sleepless night can cause you to feel more irritable and less capable of managing stress. See *Chapter 10* for more information on how to best manage your sleep. Make sure you don't use sleeping pills—they cause all sorts of problems, as described in *Chapter 12*.

EAT A HEALTHY DIET

Fueling your body with healthy, nutrient-rich foods helps you maintain your physical health, keeps your energy high, and enables you to feel your best. Experts agree that the healthiest diets are those that involve minimal intake of processed food (such as potato chips and many cereals) and high intake of fruits, vegetables, beans, whole grains, nuts, and seeds. Processed food has had mechanical or chemical operations performed to change or preserve it. They are foods that typically come in a box or bag and contain a long list of ingredients. Note that some processed foods are healthy, like tofu, frozen vegetables, and precooked whole grains. One way to help determine which processed foods are healthy is to look at the ingredients list. If the list includes ingredients you could add yourself at home (such as olive oil), then it is minimally processed. If the ingredients can only be made in a factory or laboratory (for example, hydrogenated oil or soy protein isolate), then the food is more likely to be highly processed.

The Mediterranean diet has been extensively studied and is one of the healthiest diets. It is easy to follow, focuses on the consumption of whole foods, and features seafood and plant-based eating. It emphasizes the consumption of fruits and vegetables at every meal, whole grains, beans, nuts and seeds, and fish at least twice a week. Although it is low in saturated fats, it encourages consumption of the "good fats" found in nuts and olive oil. The diet also recommends low consumption of eggs, dairy, and poultry, with rare consumption of sugar and red meat. It also focuses on socializing over meals with friends and family. Likely for all of these reasons, the Mediterranean diet has been linked to improved physical and emotional health—and longer life.

LIMIT ALCOHOL CONSUMPTION

People often ask about the risks and benefits of drinking alcohol. This is an especially important question because caregivers are at increased risk of abusing alcohol in an effort to cope with stress and other negative emotions. The current Dietary Guidelines for Americans recommends that *if* alcohol is consumed, it should be in moderation. A drink is defined as 5 ounces of wine, 12 ounces of beer that contains 5% alcohol, or 1 ounce of liquor. Moderate alcohol use is one drink per day for women and up to two drinks per day for men consumed on any single day—not intended as an average over several days. Due to age-related changes in how the body metabolizes alcohol, however, we strongly recommend no more than one drink per day for both women and men over the age of 65. In fact, some research suggests that even this amount may be too much, warning that daily consumption of alcohol may be associated with increased health risks. For all these reasons, we do not recommend that anyone start drinking alcohol to cope with stress or for any other reason. If you do drink alcohol, we recommend that you do not exceed the recommended guidelines.

What do you do if you simply enjoy the taste of beer, wine, or cocktails and you don't want to reduce the amount you are drinking? The good news is that there are now a number of non-alcoholic beers, wines, and cocktails you can buy that are actually quite tasty! Try a few and see which you like best.

MEDICAL CARE: GET IT—DON'T IGNORE IT!

Sara presses her breast firmly with her fingers. *I think this lump is bigger.* She feels it again. *I'm sure it's bigger.* She schedules an appointment with her doctor.

"You noticed this lump 4 or 5 months ago and you're just coming to see me now?" her doctor asks.

Sara swallows and responds, "Yes, I've been busy . . ."

"Breast cancer is nothing to fool around with. We have many treatments that work, but we need to catch it early."

"You're saying it's cancer?"

"I don't know. We need to do a mammogram—looks like you missed your last one—and, depending upon what it shows, perhaps a biopsy as well."

Have you missed, canceled, or not scheduled a medical appointment for yourself because you have been so focused on providing the best care to your loved one? If so, you are not alone. Many caregivers delay—or neglect altogether—treating their own health conditions. To maintain your own physical health, it is essential to make time for your annual exams and routine medical care in addition to promptly addressing any unexpected ailments that arise. If you can't remember the last time you had an annual exam, call your doctor's office now (yes, set the book down and call; you can leave a message if they are closed). It is also important to visit your doctor quickly if you have any concerns about your health. Ignoring your own physical health will only lead to larger health problems in the future.

TAKE CARE OF YOUR EMOTIONAL HEALTH

There are many things you can do to improve your emotional health and manage feelings of stress, depression, and anxiety. In fact, everything that we have already discussed to help your physical health—aerobic exercise, restful sleep, a healthy diet, and treating medical problems—will also help your emotional health. Next we discuss the importance of knowing when to seek professional help for your emotions, maintaining social connections, taking time for yourself, learning relaxation therapy, practicing meditation, and finding joy—all things that are also crucial for your physical health.

Recognize when to seek professional help for your emotions

At times, the emotions you experience may become overwhelming. Many caregivers experience such deep sadness, anxiety, or stress that they need the support and guidance of a professional to help manage these feelings. A counselor, social worker, or psychologist can suggest coping strategies to help you manage your emotions and practical skills to help you manage your responsibilities in daily life. You can also discuss existential issues related to loss and death in the context of caring for your loved one.

Sometimes people feel reluctant to request professional help even when it would be beneficial. Some people worry they will be thought of as "weak" or "crazy" if they seek professional help. Reaching out for help is nothing to be embarrassed about. Moreover, the earlier you obtain help, the sooner it can be effective.

So, how do you know if you should seek professional help? There are some signs to look for that may signal it would be beneficial. In *Chapter 8* we reviewed some common symptoms of depression and anxiety as they might present in your loved one. The same symptoms apply when considering your own mood. Review the common symptoms of depression and anxiety listed in *Chapter 8*, and if you experience two or more of these symptoms, think about obtaining professional help.

Maintain your social connections

It should come as no surprise that caring for someone with dementia is not something that can be done alone, yet the majority of caregivers report feeling alone or isolated. In *Chapter 15* we discuss in depth how to build your care team. Here we want to emphasize how important it is to maintain your social connections as a critical part of your emotional wellbeing. Studies have found that maintaining social connections is a protective factor for caregivers, increasing their resilience even in the face of multiple stressors. Finding the time to remain connected can be challenging. We recommend that you set up one or more standing weekly meetings with friends and family—maybe a half-hour walk each morning with your neighbor and a weekly cup of coffee with a friend. Limited for time? Invite friends and family to visit you at your house so you don't end up spending the bulk of your time in transit.

Take time for yourself

In *Step 5* we discuss a number of enjoyable activities that you can engage in together with your loved one and the benefits of doing so. Here we focus on some of the pleasant activities you can do on your own as a way to take care of yourself.

To start, make a list of all the things that you enjoyed before you became a caregiver. Maybe you liked to take a long bath or get a revitalizing massage or go to an exercise class. Maybe you used to read, play the piano, go jogging, do puzzles, or create artwork in your free time. (Set down the book and write your list.) Once you have made your list, think about which activities you want to keep that fit your current budget and lifestyle. Now actually schedule time to do one or more of these activities each week, for at least a half-hour. (Stop reading, open up your calendar, and add them to your schedule.) When caregivers don't schedule time for themselves, they don't take time for themselves.

Many caregivers say, "When I get everything done, then I'll do something for myself." But rarely does everything get done. You may have less time than before to do the things you enjoy, but it is vital to set aside some time to do something pleasant just for yourself.

Learn relaxation techniques

Sara looks at the clock. 12:32 AM. She will hear about her biopsy result this afternoon. She closes her eyes and rolls over, trying again for asleep. *What if I needed surgery? Who would take care of my daughter—and my father?*

Rolling onto her back, she peeks at the clock. 12:34 AM. Sighing heavily, she climbs out of bed. Sitting cross-legged on the floor, she uses the relaxation technique she learned.

Fifteen minutes later Sara is back in bed and feeling serene. She smiles inwardly at her accomplishment as sleep wraps around her.

Relaxation techniques can help you manage stress and negative emotions. Next we briefly review the techniques we teach most often: deep breathing and progressive muscle relaxation. You can also find numerous videos and audio recordings online that illustrate these methods. There are also mobile apps that provide guided relaxation and stress-reduction techniques.

Breathe deeply

Most of us take shallow breaths throughout the day. When you take shallow breaths, you may feel your chest or shoulders rise. In deep breathing, your diaphragm (the muscle between your lungs and abdomen) pushes down into your abdomen, expanding your lungs fully and making your belly rise. Breathing deeply helps you feel calm by activating your parasympathetic nervous system, the system in your body responsible for helping you to rest and relax.

The first step in practicing deep breathing is to become familiar with the feeling of taking a deep breath. It is often best to begin lying down. Pick a firm and stable spot, like the floor or a mat, and place one hand on your chest and the second on your stomach, just below the ribcage. Breathe in deeply and slowly through your nose. Do you feel the hand on your stomach rise as your stomach is pushed out? The hand on your chest should remain relatively still. Breathe out slowly through your lips and repeat up to 10 times. Once you become familiar with the feeling of deep breathing, you can do the same exercises sitting or standing.

At first, it may take effort as your body adjusts to a new way of breathing but, over time, breathing deeply will become easier and more routine. Deep breathing can be a helpful part of your daily routine. You can also use it anytime you are feeling stressed or anxious. Try setting aside 10 to 20 minutes each day for deep breathing; it can reduce chronic stress and anxiety as well as strengthen the practice so it will work better for you whenever an urgent need arises.

Relax your muscles

When we are under stress, the muscles of our body become tense. Progressive muscle relaxation teaches you how to relax your body by slowly tightening and then loosening different muscle groups while engaging in focused breathing.

To begin, sit or lie down in a comfortable position. Take several deep breaths to center yourself. Bring your awareness to a specific muscle group, such as those in your feet. Starting with your toes, contract each muscle firmly but gently, without straining, while breathing in. On the exhale, intentionally relax these muscles. Progress from your toes to your head (or your head to your toes, if you wish) until all muscles have been targeted.

Progressive muscle relaxation increases your awareness of how your body feels when it is stressed versus relaxed. This technique has been shown to be effective for lowering stress and anxiety. You can find many progressive muscle relaxation scripts and videos online; you can also use a mobile app or ask your healthcare provider for specific resources.

Practice mindfulness and other forms of meditation

Did the relaxation techniques just described remind you of mindfulness or other forms of meditation? That's because focusing on your breathing and learning to relax your muscles are fundamental elements of meditation. There are numerous books, videos, audio recordings, and websites from which you can learn more information. We've included the relevant National Institutes of Health websites under *Further resources* at the end of the book. There are also mobile apps that you can download to your phone or other device that provide guided mindfulness and meditation techniques.

RECOGNIZE THE JOYS OF CAREGIVING

Sara takes her daughter, Claire, and her father out to dinner.

"This is a nice restaurant, Sara. What's the occasion?" Jack asks.

"I heard some good news today," Sara says, smiling. "My doctor called to tell me that I am completely healthy."

"That's wonderful! Speaking of health, I want to thank you for everything you've done for *my* health—coming over here each morning to help me with my pills. I really appreciate it."

"Thanks, Dad, for saying that." *Just this little gratitude is enough to make trekking across town every morning worth it*, Sara thinks as a warm glow spreads throughout her body.

As Sara and Claire are driving home from dinner, Claire says, "I can't believe all the stories Grandpa told us tonight! I love that one when he raced a police officer in his car—and won—only to find the officer waiting for him in his driveway at home. I want to hear all of Grandpa's stories while . . ." Claire trails off.

"While he can still remember them?"

"Yes."

"That's nice. We can certainly try to spend more time with him."

"But we're so busy. And I worry about him being all alone, and not being able to drive or anything."

"O . . . kay," Sara says slowly.

"What do you think about Grandpa moving in with us?"

Sara's eyebrows rise up in surprise. "Move in with us?"

"Why not? Then you wouldn't need to race across town to give him his medicines every morning. And if he were in our house, I could help too!"

After pausing to think through several pros and cons and logistical issues, Sara says, "Claire, that is a brilliant idea! It would be great for your grandfather, much easier for me, and—absolutely—you could help too. Let's ask him about it this Sunday."

Sara smiles, knowing she will actually enjoy having more leisure time to spend with her father.

Despite many negative parts of caregiving, most caregivers are able to identify some benefits, joys, and uplifts to caring for their loved one with dementia. You may find you are gratified by your ability to provide excellent care, proud of strengths you didn't know you had, or pleased to give back to your loved one who has given of themselves in the past. You may feel grateful for the opportunity and motivation to heal past hurts. Or you may find joy in small aspects of providing care, such as a shared smile, laugh, or peaceful moment. You may also find that you are making new friends and strengthening your existing relationships through your experience providing care.

Your ability to identify positive aspects of caregiving can help reduce some of its negative aspects and enhance your wellbeing. Pause each week and consider some of the positive aspects of providing care for your loved one. Have you learned something valuable about yourself? Have you deepened your connection with your loved one? Are there other ways this experience has created an opportunity for something positive to blossom?

MORE WAYS TO CARE FOR YOURSELF

In *Chapter 15* we will discuss the important role of support groups and other resources that can also help you manage depression, anxiety, and other negative emotions while building skills needed to cope with caregiving responsibilities.

SUMMARY

Caregivers experience higher rates of emotional and physical illness. They are often so focused on taking good care of others that they put themselves last. This is particularly true for the sandwich generation caring for both aging parents and growing children. Remember, you can't pour from an empty cup. In order to care for others, you must take care of yourself. This means scheduling time for your physical and emotional health. Exercise regularly. Sleep well. Eat healthy foods. Limit alcohol intake. Get medical care. Maintain your social connections. Take time for yourself. Learn relaxation techniques. Seek professional help when needed. Look for the joys of caregiving.

Let's consider a few examples to illustrate what we learned in this chapter.

- *Your diet has never been very good and, since you started caring for your father, it has become much worse. You tend to stop at fast-food restaurants and grab anything convenient. You'd like to eat better, but you don't even know where to start.*
  - ○ Changing your diet may seem difficult, but there are some easy guidelines you can use to make healthier food choices. Reducing your intake of processed foods—those prepackaged foods with many ingredients—and increasing your intake of whole foods,

like fresh fruits and vegetables, is a good place to start. Next, try the Mediterranean diet, which involves eating fruits and vegetables at every meal, fish at least twice a week, whole grains, and "good fats" like those found in nuts and avocados. Low intake of dairy products is recommended; red meat and sugar should be consumed rarely.

- *You just don't have the time to do anything for yourself. Between getting the kids ready for school and making sure your mother is cared for, there is no time left in the day to think about what you need. You've been feeling really lousy lately, but you just can't find time to see your doctor.*

  ○ There is often so much to do each day that finding time for yourself can be hard. But it's critical that you do find some time to take care of your own physical and emotional health—or you may end up getting sick yourself! Make an appointment with your primary care provider for a checkup if you have not had one recently. Talk to them about how you've been feeling. Taking the time to care for yourself will help you provide the best care to others.

- *Maybe you're thinking, "No one understands what I'm going through. Since my husband was diagnosed with dementia, I feel embarrassed to see any of my friends. What would I tell them? They wouldn't know what to say. Plus, I don't have time to have fun. I need to focus on my husband now."*

  ○ It can be difficult to decide whether or not to reveal a diagnosis of dementia to friends and family, and it can be tempting to avoid socializing so you don't have to talk about uncomfortable things. Nevertheless, remaining social and engaged with others is important for your own physical and mental health. Find some trusted friends and family members whom you can meet with regularly, even if it is only for a half an hour a week. Ask if friends and family can come to you in order to reduce your time spent traveling. In *Chapter 15*, we will also talk about finding new people to socialize with through support groups and other activities. These experiences can offer you ways to connect with people who are going through similar experiences.

15

How do you build your care team?

Caring for a loved one with dementia is not a task that can be accomplished alone. You need a care team—and you need to build it early, immediately following a diagnosis. Your care team are the people and resources you will turn to for help in caring for your loved one—and yourself. Organizing a care team seems like an obvious idea, right? Nevertheless, survey results found that more than half of caregivers reported feeling alone or isolated, and the majority of caregivers reported wanting more support in their caregiving efforts. We all agree that it takes a village to provide the care needed for someone living with dementia. Let's explore how you can build a strong and supportive care team.

ASK FOR HELP

Martin crawls into bed after putting the dirty linens into the washer. *At least Nina is asleep,* he thinks. He glances at the clock. *3:03 AM.* He closes his eyes again, but he can't stop the whirl of thoughts rushing through his head.

How long can I keep this up? It feels like years since I've had a good night's rest.

Should I ask my son to come over more? No, he's busy—he's got his
   own life. And you can do this, Martin.
Maybe some of our friends could help out—at least the ones we have
   left. Interesting how some suddenly became "too busy" to see
   us once Nina developed dementia. No, I don't want to scare the
   others away.
Didn't you promise, "for better, for worse, for richer, for poorer, in sick-
   ness and in health"? After 60-plus years of marriage, are you going
   to quit on her now?
And what would all your relatives think? They'd say, "Oh, that Martin,
   he couldn't handle it when things got tough."
Better to simply carry on. I just don't think I've ever felt so . . . alone.

The first and sometimes most difficult step in building your
care team is reaching out and asking for help. You may feel like
you can do it alone—or you *should* do it alone—but remember: No one can do it alone. It isn't a sign of weakness or irre-
sponsibility to ask for help; on the contrary, it is a sign that you
know what you're up against and that you want to provide your
loved one with the best care possible. Often caregivers feel guilt
or shame about asking for help. If you're struggling with these
kinds of feelings, it may be time to seek professional support
to help you manage these emotions so that you will have the
courage to reach out (see *Chapters 8* and *14*). Once you do reach
out, you will likely be surprised at how eager your family and
friends are to help you. Everyone needs support when caring
for a loved one with dementia.

Part of asking for help is feeling comfortable sharing your
loved one's diagnosis with others. For those who frequently
share important events in their lives with friends, this sharing may be an easy and natural thing to do. But for those who
are more private by nature, sharing may feel awkward or difficult. You may not want to burden others with your problems.
Your loved one may be a private person and you may simply
want to respect their wishes. Or perhaps you worry that you

will be ostracized by your social group if you reveal the diagnosis. Regardless of the reason for your hesitation, some amount of sharing is necessary to build your care team so that you and your loved one can receive all of the help you need. Good friends will be supportive.

ENGAGE FAMILY AND FRIENDS

Your care team begins with those who know you best, your family and friends. If you are already caring for your loved one with another person or a small group of people, this is your *core care team*. If you are not, think about whether there are one or more people who might be able to partner with you to care for your loved one. Once your team is formed, it is helpful to meet together, with or without your loved one, to go over what kinds of tasks your loved one will need help with. Then you can decide who will be responsible for each task. Think about each team member's strengths and weaknesses, interests and skills, and location (near or far) in determining who is best suited for each task. Having these important conversations with your core care team and coming up with a care plan soon after a diagnosis is important—don't wait until there is a crisis!

In some cases, there may appear to be no core care team available. You may be the only caregiver for your loved one, and the family and friends who could assist you may not be so obvious. Either way, it is always helpful to identify additional people who can form your extended care team and offer assistance. Start by making a list of all the family members and friends of both yourself and your loved one, whether or not you think they could be part of your care team. These are usually people who already know about your loved one's diagnosis or with whom you feel comfortable sharing the information. It doesn't matter if they live close by or far away. Once you have your list, circle the names of at least three people who might be willing to help with even very small tasks. If you can circle more, that's great!

If you find yourself circling just one name, then start there. For each name circled, think about the tasks, large or small, that person might be able to do. Maybe someone on the list would be willing to stay with your loved one for an hour each week (or each month), giving you some time for yourself. Maybe someone else would be willing to accompany your loved one to an appointment. Or pick up your loved one's medications. Or drop off a meal once a month. Or help you with the laundry. Or mow your yard. Or run an errand.

Caring for an individual with dementia can also present the opportunity to make new friends who can serve as strong sources of support throughout the disease course. Joining a caregiver group and attending activities that are offered specifically for individuals with dementia and their caregivers provide opportunities to connect with others going through a similar situation. These new friends may be in a better position to understand the issues you're experiencing because they're facing many of the same challenges. They may be able to offer practical tips and suggestions about how you can manage some difficult problems, as they may have faced them earlier. And you may find it rewarding to be able to offer advice to others from lessons that you've learned during your caregiving journey.

ENLIST NEIGHBORS

"How's Nina doing?" Martin hears as he closes the mailbox. He turns around to see his neighbor walking toward him.

"Oh, she's fine, just fine," Martin replies.

The neighbor looks at Martin and then says kindly, "Remember that I took care of my father when he had dementia. It was a pretty rare day when everything was 'just fine.'"

Martin cannot help smiling as he thinks, *Here's someone who's been through this before.*

"Alright," he says, "Nina's been going through a tough patch lately, up a lot in the middle of the night."

The neighbor nods. "What can I do to help?"

Martin begins to say, "Nothing"—but catches himself and says, "You know what would really be helpful? When I need to run to the store for a few minutes to get something, I just don't feel comfortable leaving Nina alone. Do you think you could . . . I mean, would you mind . . ."

"I would be glad to come over and be with Nina while you're out. Just let me know what she likes and how she's liable to get into trouble."

"Great!" Martin says with gratitude. "With help from my son, I've got that written down. Nina will likely be just fine with you there to keep her company."

You and your loved one may have spent years building a community of friends in your neighborhood. You should consider sharing the diagnosis of dementia with your close neighbors who can offer some support and practical assistance. Neighbors can serve as an extra pair of eyes, noticing changes in your loved one that you may miss when you're away from home or if you are caring from afar. Some neighbors will be happy to visit your loved one's home, go for a walk around the neighborhood with them, or take them on an errand. Neighbors may spot your loved one wandering and be able to intervene before they become lost. Or they can help if your loved one appears confused at a local store. Especially for caregivers who live far away, having neighbors who are willing to check in on your loved one and provide you with updates can be invaluable.

FAR FROM HOME

Your care team doesn't have to consist only of family and friends who live close by. There are many things that those who live far away can help with, such as coordinate meal delivery, manage your loved one's finances online, and help research resources in your community.

Members of the care team who are not local can also plan to visit your loved one. When they are visiting, there may not be time to do everything. Make a list of priorities for the visit to ensure the most important tasks get done. It's also important for these members of the team to make time to connect with your loved one and do some relaxing and enjoyable activities during visits. See *Step 5* for specific ideas and ways to ensure that outings are successful.

Between visits, caregivers at a distance can stay in touch through phone calls and the video-chat technologies available on every smartphone. The software and calls are usually free. There are also many stand-alone video-chat technology platforms available. Distance caregivers can also send greetings and photos via email to local caregivers who can then share these messages with your loved one.

Perhaps you are the primary caregiver despite the fact that you live far from your loved one. Although more difficult, this situation can be managed as long as there is someone nearby who can help with those things that need to be done in person. The local caregiver might be a friend, neighbor, cousin, niece, or nephew who is able to take your loved one to doctors' appointments and visit their home periodically. If there are no friends or family nearby, a local geriatric care manager can play the same role; see later in this chapter for more information about these professional caregivers. Of course, another option if your loved one lives far from you and there is no one local to help is to move your loved one close to you; see *Chapter 18* for a discussion of housing options.

Lastly, it is worth pointing out one advantage of distance. When you are with someone almost every day, it can be difficult to notice small, gradual changes. That's why someone who only occasionally sees your loved one may actually be better at noticing some of the changes than you are.

SHARE INFORMATION AND ORGANIZE YOUR CARE TEAM

One way to keep track of the responsibilities of a care team is to use a shared calendar so everyone is clear about what they are doing and when. Entries may include daily tasks, such as "Stop by to make sure pills are taken," as well as appointments to doctors' offices and luncheons with friends. There are simple ways to share calendars via websites, computer programs, and phone apps. There are also several free, online shared calendars that families can use to manage their care team. In addition to calendars, these websites often include other features, such as the ability to post tasks for which help is needed, allowing team members to sign up for the tasks they can do. Consider using shared drives, secure folders, and other ways to electronically share lists of medications, phone numbers of health care providers, and any other information that multiple team members may need. Using a shared calendar, centralizing important documents, and using other organizational tools can help make caregiving easier. See *Further Resources* at the end of this book for more information.

ATTEND SUPPORT GROUPS

In addition to introducing you to new friends, support groups are an important part of your care team. They can be a source of valuable information, teach you new skills, reduce isolation, and provide a brief respite. They are nonjudgmental and can provide you with an opportunity to vent your feelings. Support groups are often divided into three broad categories—*informational, skill building*, and *emotional*—although most support groups serve overlapping functions, providing some degree of all of these things.

Informational support groups are frequently limited in duration and structured; for example, an hour each week over 8 weeks. They are usually led by an expert in dementia who is teaching information as in a classroom. Gaining education about Alzheimer's disease and dementia can increase your ability to provide care and prepare you for the challenges that lie ahead.

Skill building groups focus on teaching you a specific skill or set of skills that are useful for navigating particular caregiving challenges. These groups include an informational component, similar to that described in the previous paragraph, as well as an interactive component, where specific skills are taught and practiced. Discussion between the group leader and caregivers facilitates the learning. Skill building groups can help you improve communication, manage difficult behaviors, and cope with your emotions. Although we discuss many of these skills in this book, groups provide an opportunity for individualized training, can help you apply the training to your personal experiences, can help you to troubleshoot problems, and allow you to learn from and connect with other caregivers.

Emotional support groups are usually organized and led by a moderator who facilitates the group by welcoming everyone, making general announcements that may be of interest to all, and giving each member the opportunity to introduce themselves and talk a bit about their personal caregiving journey. These meetings are not like classes. Instead, they provide an opportunity for caregivers to share their stories and offer emotional support to one another as well as tips and suggestions from their own experiences. Emotional support groups are often ongoing and do not have a formal beginning and end.

Finding the time to attend support groups can sometimes be challenging. Perhaps you would need to leave your loved one alone to attend a support group. If this is an issue, ask the organizers of the group if they offer a concurrent session for individuals with dementia; sometimes they do, providing you with much-needed short-term respite. In addition to in-person support groups, there are also increasing opportunities to join telephone, video, and online support groups, which can remove the burdens of getting to a physical location and finding respite care for your loved one. These electronic options may be particularly attractive if you live in a rural area. (See *Further Resources* at the end of this book for more information regarding online groups.) In addition, hospitals and clinics may provide access to support groups via a video platform. Ask your health care provider if these types of services are available in your area.

Lastly, another way to build your support network is to visit a "memory café." See *Chapter 17* for more information.

CONSIDER PROFESSIONAL CAREGIVERS

Depending on the needs of your loved one, you may consider getting help from one or more professional caregivers. *Geriatric care managers* are licensed professionals specifically trained to assess, plan, coordinate, and provide services for individuals with dementia, such as exploring options for long-term care, finding community resources, facilitating discussions around sensitive topics, and coordinating with your loved one's health care providers. Their educational backgrounds may include social work, gerontology, or nursing. They can be particularly valuable in finding and coordinating local services if you are the primary caregiver and you live far from your loved one. *Visiting nurses* can come to your loved one's home to administer medications and help with other medical issues, such as wound care and routine monitoring of blood pressure or blood sugar. *Home health aides* can help with many personal care activities, such as bathing and feeding your loved one. Meal delivery services, like *Meals on Wheels*, can help by bringing nutritious meals to your loved one's door. *Homemakers* can come to the house to help with laundry, cooking, light cleaning, and similar tasks. Many communities now have senior volunteers, such as *Seniors Helping Seniors*, who can provide companionship and assistance to older adults with dementia. See *Further Resources* for more information on these topics.

USE RESPITE CARE

"What are you doing here on a Sunday, son?" Martin says as he opens the door.

"I thought I'd stop by and spend a little time with Mama."

"That's nice of you, but you can't spend all of your free time here."

"I know, but Pop, I've been thinking. Mama is having more bowel and bladder accidents. And people don't like to visit when she doesn't recognize them anymore. Maybe it's time for her to go to a program during the day."

"Day care! She doesn't need that. I can take care of your mother just fine in our home."

"I know you can. But is it the best thing for you?"

"What do you mean?"

"You're running yourself ragged. You're not getting enough sleep— and I bet you have no time for yourself."

"You think your old man can't handle it. I'm telling you, I can take care of your mother."

"Pop, I know you can. Look, it's not the best thing for Mama either. She would benefit from getting out of the house and seeing other people."

Martin sees the earnestness in his son's eyes. He hesitates, and then says, "But what do you think your aunt and our other relatives would say? They'd say I couldn't manage Nina on my own."

"And they'd be right! No one can care for someone with dementia by themselves."

We've already suggested some ways in which your care team can provide respite, such as scheduling outings with your loved one and spending time visiting with them in the home. We also suggested finding out if your loved one can attend a group while you attend a caregiver-specific group, and how you can use professional caregivers. Here we discuss respite care, in which your loved one can spend time in a program during the day or overnight if you are away.

You may have concerns about paying for these and other types of professional respite care. Although most health insurance does not cover respite care, some facilities will offer payment on a sliding scale relative to your income, so ask about such an option. Some volunteer organizations provide respite care free of charge. Medicare, Medicaid, long-term-care insurance, and military veteran benefits should be explored as potential alternative sources of payment for respite care. Financial assistance may be available through federal, state, or local organizations. See *Further Resources* for more information.

CONSIDER DAY PROGRAMS AT ADULT DAY CENTERS

Adult day centers run day programs that your loved one can go to for 1 or more days each week. These programs are usually beneficial to both you and your loved one. We usually recommend beginning with 2 days a week—frequent enough that your loved one will find it familiar. Most centers provide close monitoring of your loved one, stimulating activities, and opportunities for socialization. Most centers can also help with personal hygiene and administer medications; some provide additional services such as occupational and physical therapies. Staff qualifications differ between centers; some have nurses and a few have physicians. Because adult day centers vary widely, you should visit potential centers and ask many questions to help determine whether the center meets your unique needs. Make sure the facility is clean, warm, inviting, and free of clutter, with adequate space to accommodate activities for individuals with different needs. Consider the following questions and see *Further Resources* for additional information:

- Which stages of dementia does the program serve?
- Can they accommodate people in wheelchairs, and those with hearing and vision impairments?
- How often will my loved one be evaluated to know what their interests, abilities, and needs are?
- Will medical needs, cognitive functioning, and social skills be evaluated?
- Are examinations offered for teeth, feet, eyes, ears, and blood pressure?
- Are physicians, nurses, and other health care professionals available either onsite or on call?
- Does the center provide physical, occupational, or speech therapy? Are therapists onsite?
- Does the center dispense medications or offer medication reminders?
- What activities are offered? Are the activities flexible based on needs and interests?
- Do the staff assist with grooming, toileting, eating, showering, and toothbrushing?
- What meals and snacks are offered? Are they nutritious? (Consider sampling a meal.)
- Does the center provide support groups or other help for families?
- What is the ratio of staff to clients?
- Who are the staff and what qualifications do they have? Are volunteers used?
- Are staff members provided with dementia-specific training?
- Who owns the center? How long has it been in operation? Is the center accredited?
- What are the hours of operation? Is there a minimum number of hours that participants must attend? What are the policies regarding being tardy or absent?
- What is the daily cost? What types of payments are accepted? Is there financial aid available or a sliding scale? Are there additional costs for special services?
- Does the center offer transportation at additional cost?

OVERNIGHT RESPITE

You may need respite care for a longer period of time while you travel, care for your own physical health, take a rest from the responsibilities of caregiving, or for other reasons. In these situations, having your loved one stay overnight in a care facility for 1 or more days can be a helpful option. In addition to helping you, inpatient respite care can also benefit your loved one by providing them with some variety, giving them the opportunity to form new friendships, and allowing them to return home to a refreshed household.

EASE YOUR LOVED ONE
INTO RESPITE CARE

Although sometimes urgent matters arise, whenever possible we recommend that you ease your loved one into respite care. Think for a minute about how you would feel if you were suddenly dropped off in an unfamiliar place, without anyone you knew, and you didn't understand why you were there or where your loved ones were. Without preparation, the transition to the respite program can be confusing, anxiety provoking, and alarming to your loved one. For this reason, we recommend the following approach.

Begin by discussing the transition with your loved one. We generally recommend referring to the respite program as a "club" (for a day program), a "hotel" (for overnight respite), or another label that would be descriptive but not threatening to your loved one. Explain that you wish to visit the "club" or "hotel" to find out more about their services. Travel there with them, go inside together, and simply sit down and spend 15 to 30 minutes chatting with staff and other people. Go back the following day and spend a bit longer, perhaps an hour. At some point during that visit, mention to your loved one that you are just stepping away for a few minutes to use the bathroom, and leave your loved one engaged with staff or participating in an activity for 5 to 15 minutes. Return the next day and, after spending 10 to 15 minutes getting your loved one comfortable, mention that you need to run an errand and will be back in a few minutes. Return after 30 to 60 minutes, and continue to stay so that the whole visit is about 2 hours. Begin the following day in the same way, but this time explain that your errands might take a little while; leave your loved one there for the whole day. You have now successfully eased your loved one into respite care. Use a similar approach for transportation, going with your loved one in the van a couple of times if they don't want to go in the van without you.

BENEFIT FROM NATIONAL AND COMMUNITY ORGANIZATIONS

Many countries have national organizations dedicated to helping people with Alzheimer's disease and other causes of dementia and their caregivers. In addition to informational websites, online support groups, and telephone help lines, these organizations typically have local chapters offering numerous resources that may be in or near your community. Your local community center and faith-based groups may also offer resources for you and your loved one with dementia. See *Further Resources* for more information.

ENGAGE YOUR LOVED ONE'S DOCTOR

Lastly, your loved one's doctor should also be an important member of your care team. Depending on their specialty, training, and experience (as well as the other staff in the office), the doctor may play a major, guiding role or a supportive, minor role. Either way, the doctor and their team should always be willing to answer questions that you may have and to evaluate your loved one when you are concerned about a medical problem.

Sometimes it may appear that your loved one's doctor no longer has time for them or only wants to focus on the medical issues and not the dementia. Or perhaps their long-time doctor was superb, but you find your loved one is not getting the same care from the doctor at the facility where they are now living. We encourage you to speak up any time you feel that your loved one isn't receiving the care and attention from their doctor that they need. If speaking up doesn't improve the situation sufficiently, you might want to look for another doctor, perhaps one who focuses on dementia. Geriatricians are a good option, as are behavioral neurologists and geriatric or neuro-psychiatrists, if these specialists are available in your area.

SUMMARY

No one person can manage the demands of dementia alone. Building a strong care team early following a diagnosis is critical to your wellbeing and to providing your loved one with the best care. By reaching out to family, friends, neighbors, and professional caregivers, you can limit your burden, reduce your feelings of isolation, and create a healthier environment for you and your loved one. Your loved one's doctor should be a source of help as well. Support groups can provide you with information and important skills in addition to emotional support. Whether as a day program or overnight stay, respite care may be an invaluable resource for you. National organizations dedicated to Alzheimer's disease and dementia can also be an invaluable resource.

Let's consider a few examples to illustrate what we learned in this chapter.

- *You've been caring for your mother by yourself since her diagnosis of Alzheimer's disease. At first it felt OK, but now you're wondering how long you can keep it up. You feel tired and overwhelmed but are hesitant to ask for help. Shouldn't you be able to handle her care by yourself?*

- o No. No one can manage the numerous demands that come with caring for a loved one with dementia by themselves. It always requires help from others. Reaching out for help is not a sign of weakness—it is critical for your welfare and that of your loved one. The best time to build your care team is early after a diagnosis, but it's never too late to start. Reach out today to family, friends, and neighbors. Consider also the professional resources that are available.

• *After your husband was diagnosed with Alzheimer's disease, you both made it a point to sit down with those closest to you and talk about what you might need. You're grateful that you have friends and family members who are helping, but none of them really understand what you're going through. It's been difficult transitioning to being a caregiver. You're the only one in your social circle who has a loved one with dementia, and you often feel alone.*

- o Even when supported by friends and family, it can be difficult when those around you don't share the experience of being a caregiver to someone with dementia. Support groups provide a wonderful opportunity to meet other caregivers who are living through a shared experience. Joining a support group can give you the space to talk about similar challenges and feelings as you offer each other emotional support along with tips and strategies. National organizations with regional chapters and your local senior centers are good places to look for support groups in your area. There are also support communities available online if you have difficulty getting to a support group outside the home.

Step 5

SUSTAIN YOUR RELATIONSHIP

We began our journey in *Step 1*, gaining a better understanding of what dementia is. In *Step 2* we learned why dementia causes problems and how to manage those problems. *Step 3* showed us how medications can help—or make things worse. In *Step 4* we learned how to build our care team and how to care for the most important member of the team—you! Our goal in *Step 5* is to help you to find ways to connect with your loved one and maintain your relationship even in the face of dementia. We start by discussing why it is so important to sustain your relationship by taking the time to engage in pleasant activities with your loved one and present some general considerations for planning activities that are fun and mutually enjoyable. We then focus on some of the different experiences you can pursue to foster your connection with your loved one and continue to take pleasure in your relationship.

16

Why is it important to sustain your relationship?

Your experience of partnering with your loved one to give and receive care occurs in the context of a longstanding relationship that predates the onset of dementia. To provide the best care for your loved one, it is important to nurture this relationship. Before the dementia, you have been the child, sibling, spouse, or friend of your loved one. Changes in memory, language, behavior, and bodily function may make it difficult for you to feel connected with them. In the context of dementia, the relationship between you and your loved one will change. Sadly, many care partners, caregivers, and their loved ones often become so focused on the illness, the changes it brings, and the chores that need doing that they forget to slow down and enjoy one another's company. This loss of enjoyment can make it difficult for you and your loved one to feel connected to each other and may lead to increased depression, anxiety, frustration, and irritability for you both. In this chapter we'll discuss how to plan pleasing activities to maximize the chances that they will be successful and enjoyable for all.

RELATIONSHIPS CHANGE IN DEMENTIA

Sara looks at Jack watching television in the living room as she rinses the spinach. She cannot tell if his eyes are open or closed. She wonders what happened to the strong, competent, confident man her father was.

I'm losing him, she thinks as she wipes tears away with the back of her hands. *He's just not the same person he was before.*

"Good night," Jack says after finishing dinner. "I'm going up to bed."

"Dad, it's only 7:30. Don't you want to play cards?"

"No thanks, kid, I'm beat. I'm going to get ready for bed."

Sara listens as Jack's footsteps recede upstairs.

"How come Grandpa never wants to play cards with us anymore?"

Sara sighs before answering, "It may be too hard for him to remember which cards have gone by."

"Okay, but why is he going to bed so early?"

"I think he's bored. He has nothing to do, so he watches TV and goes to bed early."

The connection between you and your loved one continues to be important throughout the course of the dementia. Those with a strong, healthy connection generally experience less caregiver burden compared with those who lack a healthy connection. One of the best ways to remain connected is to pursue activities where you can actually have fun! Moreover, individuals with dementia display fewer behavioral problems when they spend time doing enjoyable activities with their loved ones. It may seem impossible to think that, in the face of dementia, you can actually have fun with your loved one, but it can be done. This may be one of the hardest challenges you face as a caregiver— but it is also one of the most important.

You and your loved one may also find that your relationships with others will change after a diagnosis of dementia, with some relationships remaining strong and others weakening. About one-third of people with dementia say that they have lost friends following a diagnosis—one reason that many people with dementia and their caregivers feel uncomfortable disclosing a diagnosis of dementia to friends (or even family). There are, however, opportunities to make new friends, such as those you meet at support groups.

TAKE INTO ACCOUNT CHANGING ABILITIES AND INTERESTS

Sometimes the changes that occur with dementia make it challenging or impossible for you and your loved one to do some of the things you used to do for fun. You may need to think creatively about what you can do to take pleasure in each other's company. It is important to find other enjoyable activities to take the place of old activities or your loved one may become lonely and depressed.

The first step is to select an appropriate activity. In the early stages of dementia, your loved one may still be able to do many of the same things they did before their diagnosis. But, over time, changes in memory, thinking, behavior, and bodily function may make those old activities less enjoyable and more of a struggle. In the middle stages of dementia, your loved one may require direct assistance to engage in some activities and may not be able to do others at all. In later stages, your loved one should still be able to engage in some pleasant activities, but they must be relatively simple and require fewer choices. With a little creativity and thought, you will be able to modify old activities to fit new skill levels or find appropriate new activities for changing abilities and interests throughout the disease course.

To start, think of all the things your loved one was interested in before their diagnosis of dementia. What were their hobbies? What did they do for work? What did you do together? Then brainstorm ways to modify old activities as needed to fit new skills. For example, maybe you used to play bridge with your loved one until it became too difficult for them to remember trump. Now it might be relaxing to sit together and enjoy each other's company while playing solitaire together or simply sorting cards into categories.

There are also opportunities to engage in new activities. Perhaps your loved one never showed an interest in artistic expressions, like drawing or painting. Now may be the time to explore painting by numbers or visiting a museum to see if one of these activities is something that you can both enjoy.

TAKE THE LEAD

As we discussed in *Step 2*, your loved one may have more difficulty initiating activities and conversations because of changes that are taking place in the brain. They may have lost some of their initiative and "get up and go." This doesn't mean that they aren't interested in or capable of participating in activities; it just means that it may be up to you to take the lead in planning the activity and encouraging them to become involved.

Discuss with your loved one what they would enjoy or offer several suggestions and let them choose. If they cannot decide, take the lead and choose the activity. Place planned activities on a calendar so your loved one is aware of the plan and can look forward to upcoming events. Use pictures on the calendar if they can no longer read. Keeping your loved one aware of their schedule can also reduce anxiety and stress about participating in these events.

PLAN AHEAD

Determined to have some fun with her father, Sara is driving with him to a pottery collection at the museum and then to a hockey exhibit at the sports arena.

Traffic is terrible, Sara thinks as she taps the steering wheel. *I can't believe I forgot about the bridge construction.*

It's 4:30 when they finally pull into a parking spot.

"We're in luck! The museum closes at 5," Sara says as she hurries off to purchase tickets.

A few minutes later she returns, looking crestfallen.

"They won't sell us tickets because it's less than 30 minutes before closing," Sara says. "But let's catch the hockey exhibit. The arena is open till 7."

"Riiiiight!" Jack says, showing enthusiasm, but yawning.

They drive across town, arriving at the arena around 5:30.

"Well, this will be fun, right, Dad?"

Sara looks over to find her father fast asleep. *I forgot he always naps at this time*, she thinks.

In addition to taking the lead in deciding the activity, it can be helpful to plan out the details ahead of time. For example, let's consider an activity outside the home. You may want to plan out the easiest way to get there: whether you will use public transportation, drive in your own car, take a taxi, or use a rideshare app. It can be helpful to look up parking options in advance. (If parking is remote, is there a shuttle?) Look at a map of the facilities to identify family restrooms, wheelchair accessibility, and places to eat and drink. You may want to know the policies regarding bringing snacks with you. Some facilities have wheelchairs you can borrow or special devices to help you navigate the facility (such as audio devices at museums that orient you to the material you are looking at). Some museums will have days and times when admission is free. You may also be able to get free passes to certain facilities and events through your local library, senior center, or other organizations. Taking the time to plan your visit to a new location before you go can help reduce some of the anxiety you both may feel about visiting a new place and make your visit more enjoyable.

START SMALL

If you are trying to do a new activity or an activity you haven't done in a while, it can be helpful to start small. For example, instead of trying to go out for a full day, try a half a day or even just a half an hour to start. If that goes well, you might try to expand the amount of time you engage in the activity. Similarly, instead of traveling far from home, start by sticking to activities that are close. Once you are successful with these small activities, you can venture further and try to do more. Your successes and failures will teach you how to tackle new activities in the future.

CONSIDER TIME OF DAY

You may have already noticed that there are some times of the day when your loved one is more alert and active than others. It can be helpful to pay attention to those times so you can plan activities during them. Many individuals with dementia seem to do better in the late morning or early afternoon and can experience an increase in problems as the late afternoon and evening approaches (see the discussion of *sundowning* in *Chapter 9*). Some individuals may have fluctuations in alertness and arousal throughout the day, which can make it more challenging to plan activities, and you may need to do your best and try a couple of different times of day to see what works for you both. If you are planning an activity outside the house (such as going to a museum or movie), you may want to plan your visit not only at a time of day that works well for your loved one but also at a time of day or day of the week that is less crowded to avoid overstimulation.

GO WITH THE FLOW

There may be times when you have planned a wonderful activity, giving careful thought about what to do and when to do it, and it still does not go the way you thought it would. Perhaps your loved one refuses to engage in the activity. Maybe they start doing the thing you set out to do but then become distracted and express interest in another activity, or decide halfway through that they want to stop. Perhaps you have lovingly planned a new activity and—to your dismay—they clearly don't like it or are not interested in it. Experiences like these can be disappointing, but it is important to go into all activities with an open and flexible mind. Don't set your heart on one specific activity. Be prepared to "go with the flow." If you need to leave someplace because your loved one isn't enjoying themselves or is having trouble behaving properly, don't fight it; just leave. It may be helpful to have a backup plan or a plan for how to leave somewhere you are if things don't seem to be working out. For example, purchase aisle movie and theater tickets so it will be easy to leave in the middle if you need to. The most important thing is to focus on enjoying your time with your loved one, even if things don't go exactly as planned.

BE IN THE MOMENT

Jack moves up and down the sidelines, yelling words of encouragement to his granddaughter and her teammates.

"That was a great game you played," Jack says as they sit down to lunch. "I haven't had so much fun in years."

"Thanks for coming and cheering, Grandpa!"

"Of course! I still remember picking you up from soccer practice when you were little," Jack says.

He's smiling, Sara notices, *for the first time in weeks.*

Many of us have the idea that activities need to be unique, special, expensive, or outside of our usual daily routines to be enjoyable. Don't forget that there are many simple, free activities that may be perfect for your loved one and also fun for the whole family. Watching local sports events, doing jigsaw puzzles, swaying to music on the radio, going for a walk, and feeding the ducks are just some activities that may not sound exciting but can be enjoyed by all when you focus on each moment.

DON'T GIVE UP

Don't get discouraged if you set out to do something enjoyable with your loved one and it doesn't turn out the way you planned. Keep trying! Even if one activity doesn't work out, there are so many others you can try. Every experience is an opportunity to learn something new about your relationship with your loved one. One day may not go as planned, but the next just might. Scheduling pleasant activities in dementia is a moving target—the most important thing is to keep moving!

SUMMARY

Despite the challenges of dementia, it is important to continue to have fun with your loved one and nurture your relationship. Engaging in pleasant activities is a great way to remain connected. These activities can also help to reduce behavioral problems, boost mood, and even improve functioning in your loved one. Engaging in activities with your loved one can also help reduce burden and stress on you. Although your loved one may have trouble doing some of the things they enjoyed before their dementia, there are a variety of activities that they can still participate in. Some activities may be variations on things they used to enjoy and others may be entirely new. We encourage you to take time to engage in pleasant activities with your loved one on a regular basis.

Let's consider a few examples to illustrate what we learned in this chapter.

- *You used to play chess with your loved one every evening, but they are no longer able to remember the moves. Instead of being enjoyable, playing chess has become frustrating and unpleasant.*
  - As dementia progresses, your loved one will find it difficult to do some of the things they used to do for fun. Because of this difficulty, old hobbies and interests may become unpleasant. One option is to find ways to modify a favorite old activity.

For example, instead of playing chess, just being together and moving the pieces around on the board may be enjoyable. Or try a simpler game, like checkers. You can also try new activities that your loved one wasn't previously interested in. Perhaps they would now enjoy drawing, painting, or sculpting chessmen. Sometimes dementia presents an opportunity to find new interests and ways of having fun that weren't considered before.

- *You took your loved one to a movie, but it did not go well. The theater was crowded, your loved one was uncomfortable in their seat, and you had to step over 10 people to go to the bathroom in the middle of it. You're not going to try something like that again.*

  o It can be difficult when you try to do something fun with your loved one and it doesn't go well. But once you are back home—calm, relaxed, and recovered—you can look back, figure out what went wrong, and use what you learned for the next time. Maybe you learned that you need to go to matinees during the week when it is less crowded. Maybe you need to select a theater with more comfortable seats. Maybe you simply need to sit at the end of a row, toward the back of the theater, just in case you need to leave early (and maybe if you speak to the manager ahead of time they can even reserve those seats for you, or choose a theater with seats that can be reserved online).

- *You would like to do fun activities with your loved one, but with all the cooking, cleaning, washing, and toileting you're doing 24 hours a day—not to mention all the doctors' appointments—you simply don't have time.*

  o We know you have numerous demands on your time and it can be stressful to even think of adding one more. However, it is critical to put the chores aside for a time and have some fun with each other—studies show you will be a better caregiver if you do so! In addition to helping you remain connected, engaging in pleasant activities can reduce behavioral problems, boost mood, and improve your loved one's ability to perform activities of daily living. It can also help relieve some of the stress and burden you may feel as a caregiver, lift your own mood, and promote your health and wellbeing.

17

What are some ways to sustain your relationship?

There are many activities you can enjoy with your loved one to help sustain your relationship—too many to list them all! The ones you choose should depend on your unique interests, how much time you have, the activities you have access to, and many other personal factors. Don't forget to consider new activities in addition to your old favorites.

VISIT A MEMORY CAFÉ

Memory cafés are a place where you and your loved one with dementia can go together and be welcomed by others. Many offer an educational talk. Others focus on activities, from crafts and painting to singing and dancing. They are not a place to drop your loved one off—they are places where you can enjoy being together with your loved one. Search the internet for "memory café near me" and you may find one close to you.

MUSEUMS

A visit to a museum can be a wonderful way to connect with your loved one, as we've mentioned in *Chapter 16*. Different exhibits can stimulate dialog about what you are seeing in the moment and prompt your loved one to share personal stories from their past. Visiting a museum can also be a nice way to socialize and meet new people. Many museums have specific programs for individuals with dementia. Contact your local museum or look on their website for more information. If you find that you and your loved one enjoy the museum, consider a yearly membership—that way you can go as often as you like and you won't feel that you have to stay longer than you want to in order to "get your money's worth."

General suggestions as you prepare to visit a museum (or similar place) include avoid rushing, focus on only one room or exhibit per visit, and ask questions to facilitate discussion and engagement with the material. One museum suggests five steps designed to enhance your experience:

1. Observe the work of art without speaking.
2. Describe the work of art, asking questions such as, "What do you see in this painting?"
3. Interpret the work, thinking about the artist's intention and the historical context.
4. Connect the work of art to your own life and experience: share your personal opinions and relevant stories.
5. Summarize your thoughts about the work.

If these steps seem too involved, don't bother with them—they're just a suggestion. Visit the museum and talk about whatever comes to mind in whatever way you wish.

PERFORMING ARTS

Martin looks over at Nina nervously as the opening measures of
the sonata are played.

Halfway through the piece, Nina says loudly, "I have to go." Several
people turn to look at them.

Putting a smile on his face to cover his disappointment, he helps
her stand. "Excuse us, pardon us," he whispers again and again
as they move down the row and into the aisle.

"Never again will we go to the symphony," Martin tells their son
the next day.

"Pop, the important thing is that you gave it a try. So, it didn't work
out. Big deal. Try something different next time."

The following week Nina is sitting on the couch with her eyes
closed. Martin lowers the needle down on his old record player.

She opens her eyes as the music starts:

> *East of the sun and west of the moon,*
> *We'll build a dream house of love, dear.*

Nina begins tapping her feet. Martin sits next to her, holding
her hand.

> *Just you and I, forever and a day.*
> *Love will not die, we'll keep it that way.*

Nina is trying to stand. Martin helps her up, and they hold each
other tight, swaying to the music.

In bed that night, Martin listens to Nina's steady breathing. *You
did it*, he thinks. *You got that feeling back—at least for a little
while.* He becomes aware his pillow is damp. *What are you crying about, Martin? You should be happy.* But he knows why he's
crying. He had forgotten how nice it is to spend time together
with Nina as a couple, rather than as a caregiver and a person
with dementia.

Attending the theater to see plays, symphonies, ballets, or con-
certs can be fun for everyone. The theater encourages dialog

about the event as well as stimulating past memories and stories. Some performances are more passive, such as when you sit and observe a play or a symphony, whereas others are more active, such as when there is music where you can clap your hands, move your feet, or sing along. Consider both new performances as well as familiar plays and musical selections from your loved one's past. One special symphony program geared toward individuals with dementia and their caregivers found that the program improved alertness, engagement, mood, sense of community, and feelings of acceptance for the person with dementia. It also improved interactions between the person with dementia and their caregivers.

MOVIES

Watching movies with your loved one can be enjoyed as an outing or in the home. For individuals with dementia, it can be particularly enjoyable to watch a favorite movie from the past. Don't feel that need to watch the entire movie—just enjoy as much in one sitting as works for your loved one. You can also watch short clips of a chosen movie on the internet and use those clips to open up a discussion. In addition to watching movies at home from the usual sources, don't forget that most libraries have large selections of old movies that you can borrow and bring home or download for free.

When going out to the movies, daytime matinees are usually uncrowded and may be easier than other times. Some small, local cinemas have "sing-alongs" to musicals from the past that your loved one might enjoy. A few cinemas even have programs specifically designed for individuals with dementia and their caregivers. Search the internet to see if there is such a program near you.

MUSIC

There are many ways to incorporate music into your life. For those with dementia, music has the advantage that it is always "in the moment." Memory is not generally necessary to enjoy music. Whether passively listening, clapping your hands, moving your feet, or singing with your loved one, music can be an enjoyable activity that fosters closeness, connection, and wellbeing.

Play music your loved one finds enjoyable. Use music to set the tone. Relaxing music can be used to soothe, whereas more upbeat tunes can be used to activate, boosting mood and energy. Encourage dancing, clapping, and singing. As we discussed in *Chapter 9*, once you've found some music that your loved one enjoys, consider making some playlists with your phone, computer, compact disc (CD), or cassette tape collection. Not sure how to do this with your vinyl records? Enlist your tech- or music-savvy friends and family to help.

If your loved one previously played a musical instrument, they may be able to enjoy playing into the later stages of disease, even as other abilities fade. For individuals who have never played music, it can be fun to make music with handheld instruments, sing, or perhaps pretend to conduct an orchestra.

Lastly, you don't even need an outside source of music. You can sing your own songs together or make up songs to sing to your loved one as you complete tasks (like bathing or dressing) to make the task more enjoyable and less threatening. Singing to an individual with dementia during care situations has been shown to reduce problem behaviors and enhance communication.

ARTS AND CRAFTS

"What's all this, son?" Martin asks.

"I found some old arts and crafts supplies," he says as he carries two large shopping bags through the front door, "and I thought that you and Mama might want to use them together."

"Hi, Mama," he says as he sets down the bags in the kitchen and gives his mother a hug. He begins pulling materials out of the bags. Soon the kitchen table is covered with construction paper, glue, popsicle sticks, pieces of felt, markers, yarn, beads, old buttons, and scraps of fabric.

"Now wait a second, son," Martin begins. "I appreciate the thought, but your mother and I don't like this childish stuff."

"Come on, Pop, just give it a try."

Martin opens his mouth to respond, but then notices that Nina has picked up a button in one hand and a piece of felt in the other. She places them carefully on the construction paper, then looks up at Martin.

"Very nice, honey," Martin says, smiling in spite of himself. "I bet you do this at the day program—the club you go to—don't you?"

Nina smiles in response as she reaches for some yarn and a popsicle stick.

Engaging in arts and crafts can provide a way for individuals with dementia to express themselves, make independent decisions, gain a sense of accomplishment, and help keep motor skills strong. Consider painting, drawing, creating cards, scrapbooking, making collages, and coloring books. In fact, it seems like everywhere you turn these days you can find adult coloring books with themes ranging from designs to daisies to dinosaurs. Inherent in this relatively new adult pastime is a belief in the emotional benefits of creating art for everyone. There has even been some research to suggest coloring reduces anxiety for individuals of all ages.

You may need to help your loved one begin a project by demonstrating or verbally guiding them. Consider safety issues when doing arts and crafts; use safety scissors, nontoxic glues and paints, etc. You may find that larger tools are easier for your loved one to manipulate. One nice part of arts and crafts is that you don't need to finish the project, nor does it need to look any certain way—it is the activity that is important, not the end product. The creations can serve as a source of conversation. You might want to use a wall or shelf to display the works of art as a reminder of the time you enjoyed together. Have fun creating!

EXERCISE

We discussed in *Chapters 8* and *14* that exercise is good for the brain and can benefit both you and your loved one by improving mood and reducing problematic behaviors in dementia. Here we emphasize that exercise can also be an enjoyable activity to do together, enhancing your relationship.

Walking is one of the best exercises to do because it is free and generally well tolerated. It also allows for conversations, running errands, and connecting with nature. Stretching, Pilates, and tai chi can also be done with your loved one. Exercise classes, such as those for dance, yoga, and water aerobics, have the added benefit of increasing socialization with others and promoting new friendships. Many hospitals and medical centers offer exercise classes specifically for seniors, including those with dementia. Explore opportunities for fitness at your local YMCA or community center. Some malls offer free indoor walking programs for seniors that can be an option for you and your loved one in cold weather. It is important for both you and your loved one to check with your doctors before beginning any new exercise program, but with all the options available for exercise, you should be able to find something that works for you. See *Further Resources* for more information.

NATURE

Connecting with nature can be another enjoyable pastime for you and your loved one. Walking in a local park or a path through the woods can provide exercise while you experience natural beauty. Even spending time passively outside in a garden has been shown to reduce behavioral symptoms in individuals with dementia. Gardening, bird watching, apple picking, and visiting a farm to see the animals are other nature activities that you can enjoy doing together.

SPAS, SALONS, AND BARBER SHOPS

Many people enjoy a visit to a spa, salon, or barber shop—and it might be something you would take pleasure in doing with your loved one. It can be a fun and relaxing activity to have one's nails professionally trimmed, buffed, and painted. Or to have one's face shaved with a rich warm lather and a straight-edge razor. Most people love a massage, which can be as vigorous or light as one prefers. And everyone likes a nice haircut.

PHYSICAL INTIMACY

Greet your loved one with a hug. Offer a hand on the shoulder or a pat on the back to communicate tenderness or pride. Hold hands while taking a walk, watching a performance, or just relaxing. For spouses and couples, sexual intimacy that includes kissing, touching, and intercourse is often an important aspect of the relationship.

The importance of physical intimacy as a way to foster your relationship is often overlooked and underappreciated. Research suggests that physical intimacy is particularly important for individuals with dementia as language abilities decrease and reciprocal communication through physical touch becomes one of the few ways to remain connected.

TOUCH

A caring touch can improve blood pressure, pain, mood, and outlook. For individuals with dementia, touch has also been shown to reduce anxiety and behavioral problems. Touch stimulates the release of a hormone called oxytocin, the so-called love hormone associated with empathy, trust, and relationship-building. There are many forms of touch that you can incorporate into your interactions with your loved one. Everyday touches can include pats on the arm, holding hands, giving a hug, and brushing hair. You might also want to try more directed, conscious touches such as a back massage or foot rub.

It should be remembered that not everyone experiences touch the same way. Touch could be unwelcomed by some individuals with dementia. Obtaining verbal consent to touch is one way to ensure that the touch you are offering is wanted. Sometimes obtaining verbal consent can be difficult and other nonverbal signals of consent may be sought, such as your loved one reciprocating the touch, turning toward the touch, making eye contact, displaying decreased tension, as well as making sounds or facial expressions or showing other signs of feeling calm, comfort, and pleasure. With consent, touch can be an enjoyable and easy way to remain connected to your loved one.

MEANINGFUL ACTIVITIES

"Let me get this straight," Jack says. "A doctor wants me to speak to medical students about having dementia? I can't even spell 'dementia'!"

"That doesn't matter," Sara says. "They want you to explain what it has been like for you to have memory problems, to have left the stove on, to stop driving . . . they just want you to tell your story."

"Tell my story? Well, that I can do!"

Sara smiles to herself, so pleased that she has found an activity she can do with her father that has brought some meaning back into his life.

For healthy individuals, feeling that one has purpose in life reduces the risk of developing Alzheimer's disease and serves as a protective factor against cognitive decline. For those with dementia, a feeling of purpose can reduce depression and increase satisfaction in life. As a caregiver, you can help your loved one find meaningful activities, which can give them purpose. You can also participate in and enjoy these activities with them, boosting meaning in life for you both.

One such activity is participation in research. In our experience, caregivers and their loved ones find that participating in research provides purpose, allowing them to help their community and future generations through contributing to science and potential new treatments for dementia. See the next section in this chapter for more information about participating in research.

Another meaningful activity is participation in volunteer programs and support groups to educate people about dementia. Some universities have programs that pair individuals with dementia with health care professionals in training. These programs can help trainees better understand the experience of having dementia, improve their communication skills, and foster enthusiasm for career opportunities treating older adults. See *Further Resources* for more information.

You and your loved one may also enjoy volunteer work unrelated to dementia, such as working at a soup kitchen. There are many ways to nurture purpose, meaning, and joy in life in the face of dementia.

CONSIDER RESEARCH

Many individuals with dementia appreciate the ability to give back by donating their time to research or advocacy, gaining a sense of purpose through their efforts to help advance the science of dementia and help future generations. There are many different types of research that you and your loved one can become involved in, including clinical trials of new medications and diagnostic methods, studies of non-pharmacologic treatments such as memory aids and physical exercise, and investigations to determine the best approaches for supporting individuals with dementia and their loved ones in the community. Some studies require only a brief commitment—as short as an hour or two—whereas others will follow you and your loved one over months or years. There are several ways to find out about research opportunities that may be right for you, including Alzheimer's Disease Research Centers funded by the National Institutes of Health and Trial Match at the Alzheimer's Association. See *Further Resources* for more information about getting involved in research.

SUMMARY

There are many activities that you can enjoy with your loved one. Visiting museums, attending the theater, watching movies, and listening to music are just a few. You may both enjoy having a massage, strolling on a nature walk, or filling in an adult coloring book—even if you never pursued such pastimes before. Exercise is good for everyone and is a wonderful way to spend time with your loved one. Most people enjoy the touch and warmth of human contact and, for couples, sexual intimacy can be an important aspect of your relationship. Lastly, participating in meaningful activities—including research, advocacy, and providing support to others—can provide an important sense of purpose in life for you and your loved one.

Let's consider a few examples to illustrate what we learned in this chapter.

- *I'm interested in trying arts and crafts with my father, but I don't know which activity he'd like best. How do you choose?*
  - Have fun exploring a different activity each week. Try painting by numbers one week, adult coloring books the next, collages

or scrapbooking after that, followed by sculpting with clay, or anything else you would like to try. Get inspiration from books, friends, and the internet. Just give each activity a few days before you move on to the next. Everything is a bit more difficult the first time you do it.

- *I think my mother might enjoy holding hands when we walk but I feel a little awkward about doing it. She doesn't recognize me anymore. How would I know if that's what she wants?*
  - Not everyone wants a comforting touch, such as holding hands, but most people do. If your loved one understands language, simply ask if they would like to hold hands. If they don't understand language, you can gently take their hand in yours. If they pull away, they are telling you that they don't want to hold hands, at least at that time. If they leave their hand in yours, look at their facial expression. Are they more relaxed or tense? Do they look happier or sadder? These are clues to help you know if they are enjoying your touch.

Step 6

PLAN
FOR THE FUTURE

In *Steps 4* and *5* we discussed the importance of caring for your-self, building your care team, and sustaining your relationship with your loved one. In this last step we discuss the issues that are important to consider as you plan for the future. Dementia is a progressive disease and eventually your loved one will need help making decisions about their work life, medical care, financial management, and housing. With a little bit of work and planning, you and your care team will be there to help with these transitions. In the last chapter we discuss the eventual death of your loved one, which considerations are important for its planning, and how you can plan for your own future afterward. We acknowledge that these issues can be difficult, sensitive topics and that many of these issues may be relevant in the distant future. We have found, however, that planning for these transitions far in advance is the best way both to ease the burden of these decisions and to ensure that your loved one is able to participate in planning for their own future as much as possible.

18

How to plan for the progression of dementia

Dementia is a progressive disease: Your loved one's ability to make decisions will diminish over time as problems with memory and thinking increase. For this reason, the mild stage of dementia is usually the best time to begin planning for the issues that will arise in the moderate to severe stages. In this chapter we present a number of important issues to consider when planning for the future, including working, health care, finances, and housing.

PLAN EARLY AND INVOLVE YOUR LOVED ONE

In the mild stage, your loved one is usually capable of being involved in many decisions that will impact their future, so try to include them in future planning as much as possible. Give them the opportunity to make their wishes known. Going through transitions with your loved one later is usually easier when they've been involved in the decision-making process from the start. It can also lessen or prevent disagreements that might otherwise arise in the future when care team members express different opinions about what your loved one would have wanted if they were more able to express their opinion.

WORKING

Your loved one may still be working at the time of their diagnosis. Should they stop? It is usually good for your loved one to continue working as long as possible, provided there are no safety concerns. Working can provide your loved one with structure, intellectual stimulation, social opportunities, as well as purpose and meaning. Jobs that are usually fine to continue involve making things without power tools such as crafts, artwork, flower arranging, and knitting. Working in a store where your loved one can go at their own pace and there is always someone around to help may also be fine. However, jobs that involve power tools, chemicals, or other hazardous equipment or materials are not recommended for the person with dementia, even when they have been doing the same job for many years. Changes in memory and thinking may make your loved one unable to follow the appropriate procedures to keep themselves and others safe. Similarly, jobs that involve the supervision and care of others, such as watching children at a daycare center or performing complex care for adults, are not recommended. Jobs that involve financial management and independent decision-making, such as running a business alone or managing the assets of others, pose financial risks both to the person with dementia and to others. Jobs that involve memory, judgment, and reasoning and those that directly affect people's lives, such as clinical and legal professions, usually need to be stopped. You can serve as a source of support as your loved one makes decisions about work and transitions from working to retirement. You can also help them find other activities that can fill the time they once spent working.

MEDICAL/LEGAL ISSUES

A time will come when you need to make decisions regarding your loved one's health care. Three documents to consider when planning for future healthcare are:

- a *living will*, also known as an *advance directive*
- a *health care proxy*, also known as p*ower of attorney for health care* or *health care power of attorney* and
- a *Do Not Resuscitate order (DNR)*

If your loved one does not have these documents prepared already, we encourage you to begin discussing them soon after their diagnosis, when your loved one will be best able to clearly articulate their wishes.

Living will

A living will is a document that allows your loved one to state what kind of medical care they would want if they were not incapacitated and could make their own health care decisions, including what types of life support efforts are acceptable. Examples include whether or not they would want cancer chemotherapy, major surgery, or attempts made to restart their heart. It is never too soon to complete a living will; it is a valuable tool for everyone, not just those with dementia (you should do yours, too). Note that the laws regarding living wills vary state by state, so you should check to ensure that your loved one's living will is valid for where they are living. Although a living will can stand alone, it is usually combined with a health care proxy.

Health care proxy

"How were things at the hospital? Is your friend OK?" Sara asks.
"No," Jack responds. "I think he's dying."
"Oh, Dad," Sara says, giving him a hug.

"Thanks. I can't believe I'm going to lose him. But you know what the worst part was?"

She shakes her head.

"While my friend was in a coma three feet away, his children were arguing about what should be done. 'Should we pull the plug? Should we keep him alive and hope he'll wake up?' It was awful."

"Didn't he make his wishes known ahead of time?"

"Well, he thought so. But I can see how different people might interpret what he said differently."

"Didn't he have a living will or appoint one of his children to be health care proxy?"

"No, I'm sure he thought it wasn't necessary. I didn't think so either, until today."

A health care proxy is a document that names the individual who will be responsible for making medical and other health care decisions for your loved one should they not be able to make these decisions themselves. A health care proxy designates a specific person to make all decisions about health care and end-of-life care, including the ability to refuse treatment. The living will typically provides the health care proxy with instructions that guide their decision-making. Decisions that a health care proxy might make include choosing between different health care providers, selecting between different types of treatment, and determining levels of care. Examples include which doctor or hospital to go to, whether to undergo aggressive versus palliative (comfort-only) treatment, and when placement outside the home is appropriate. The health care proxy goes into effect when a clinician determines that your loved one no longer has the capacity to make health care decisions on their own.

Do Not Resuscitate order (DNR)

The Do Not Resuscitate order (DNR) is a specific request not to have an intervention if your loved one's heart or breathing stops. When signed by a physician, it will prevent aggressive resuscitation measures such as chest compression and breathing tubes. If desired, it should be requested by your loved one if they have the capacity to make their health care decisions, or by the health care proxy if they do not.

FINANCIAL/LEGAL ISSUES

Take care of legal issues related to finances early while your loved one still has the capacity to make financial decisions. Some of the financial issues and documents to review with an attorney include:

- *A will*
- *Estate planning*
- *Power of attorney* and
- *Trusts*

Wills and estate planning

A will is a simple document that names the person who will manage your loved one's estate and the beneficiaries of that estate after they die. In addition to a will, estate planning should also include plans for financial coverage of long-term care costs, such as the cost of in-home care, assisted living, nursing homes, and other expenses associated with declining health. Long-term care insurance is one option worth exploring to help cover long-term care expenses. Other options for long-term care needs include using a reverse mortgage, opening a health savings account, and exploring veterans benefits for those eligible. Attorneys, accountants, and estate specialists can be enlisted to assist you as you explore the options for financial planning.

Power of attorney and trusts

A power of attorney is an important document that allows your loved one to name an individual to make legal and financial decisions in the event that they are not able to make them for themselves. The person designated as power of attorney is able to take over management of real estate, tangible property, investments, bank accounts, business interests, individual retirement account assets, and taxes. You and your loved one may also consider having a living trust document, which is another legal document that allows your loved one to designate a specific individual to control those things listed in the trust, separate from what the power of attorney is able to control. In other words, the power of attorney cannot control anything in a living trust, unless they are also designated as a trustee. A living trust allows your loved one to be specific in their wishes for how items in the trust are governed and can be useful when there are specific items your loved one wants to ensure are handled in certain ways or specific persons your loved one wants to manage different pieces of their estate. You should explore both of these options with the professionals involved in assisting your loved one with financial planning.

OTHER FINANCIAL ISSUES

Talking to your loved one about finances can be challenging, but not talking about this important topic can create very serious problems later on. Declines in memory and thinking will make it difficult for your loved one to manage their finances independently.

Scams, con artists, and poor judgment

"Thirteen thousand!" Sara exclaims when she sees Jack's credit card bill. "Save the children, save the planet, save the whales, save the ozone . . ."

"That's an important one," Jack interjects.

"Maybe, but I'm not sure that all of these charities are legitimate . . . Here's one that billed you twice in the same day! What credit card is this, anyways?"

"I got it in the mail. It's interest-free!"

Sara looks at the bill. "No, the interest was only free for the first month. Then it became 37.5%! And you've only been paying off the minimum."

"But I haven't missed a payment!"

Sara closes her eyes and thinks, *It's not his fault he has dementia. Don't yell at him. It's not his fault he has dementia* . . .

Over the next few weeks, Sara worked out a system to help Jack avoid telemarketers and possible scams. She entered all of his friends, doctors, and other contacts in his cellphone. Then she turned on the setting to "silence unknown callers." Each morning before she leaves for work, she also switches off the ringer on her landline, turning it back on when she returns home in the evening.

It is unfortunate that in today's society there are individuals who use telephone, postal mail, email, the internet, and sometimes in-person solicitation to prey on older individuals with cognitive impairment. We have treated many patients who have lost thousands of dollars to such scams and con artists. In addition to discussing this possibility with your loved one so that they are forewarned, we recommend that you work with their bank and credit card companies to set up limits on how much can be spent at any one time or without additional authorization from you. Your loved one might also use poor judgment and make an expensive purchase they really cannot afford. One strategy is to set your loved one up with a separate bank account containing a small amount of money and a credit card with a low credit limit (that will not automatically go up over time). This strategy will allow them to continue their day-to-day shopping but not purchase expensive items or give away large sums of money.

Obtain permission now

Ensure now that one or more members of the core care team (whether near or far away) has written permission from your loved one to receive their medical and financial information. Share paper or electronic copies of financial and legal documents, lists of medications, phone numbers of health care providers, and so on with appropriate members of your care team. Using a secured, shared folder or drive where all items are organized can be helpful.

Work together to manage finances

Management of daily finances will become more difficult over time for your loved one, including routine bill paying, annual tax preparation, and investments. Knowing the details of their finances is essential. You should discuss what accounts they have open, usernames and passwords of electronic records, and the location of all physical documents related to finances. You need to know enough about your loved one's finances to feel confident that you can take over their management when needed.

One way to ease the transition to managing your loved one's finances is to work together as a team for as long as your loved one is able to participate. In this way, your loved one is able to show you their system and gain confidence in your ability to take over while retaining a sense of partnership in financial management. You can start by checking to make sure your loved one's checkbook is balanced and their bills are being paid on time. You may also decide to get outside help from a financial advisor for assistance with the more complex task of managing investments.

HOUSING

Even if your loved one is able to remain at home for years following their diagnosis of dementia, you'll want to begin to consider their housing needs and options as soon as possible. You may consider putting supports into place inside the home to help them remain there longer. Or you may want to look into moving your loved one from their home (or your mutual home) to an environment that can provide more support. Even if years away, it's important to start thinking about these issues now so you can avoid a crisis when the inevitable need for additional support inside or outside the home arises.

Remember that dementia progresses. Although your loved one may be able to function in their home with just a few supports from you and your care team for some period of time, they will likely need to move to a place that can provide greater care in the future. In *Chapter 15* we discuss how you and members of your care team can help to enable your loved one to remain at home as long as possible. Next we review alternate housing options available to your loved one.

How do you know it's time for a move?

You may be wondering how you will know when your loved one is ready to move to another level of care. There are some signs that suggest it is time to consider a move. Perhaps the most important is concern about your loved one's safety in their current home. Leaving the stove on, wandering, and forgetting to take medications regularly may all be signs that your loved one needs more care. It may be time for a move if your loved one is becoming physically aggressive, violent, or sexually inappropriate or is frequently incontinent of bowel or bladder. Increasing medical needs and mobility issues are other factors that can signal that it's time for a transition to a facility. For example, a wife caring for her husband who cannot walk may no longer be able to safely bring him to the bathroom, posing a fall risk for them both. As safety issues, problematic behaviors, and incontinence increase, most caregivers become more exhausted, frustrated, distressed, resentful, or frightened, and may no longer be able to provide the best care for their loved one.

Don't forget to discuss your options with your loved one's health care providers. These trusted individuals can provide their own assessment about your loved one's care needs and help guide your decision-making.

Assisted living

Assisted living facilities are state-regulated agencies that provide 24-hour care that includes a combination of personal and health care services for individuals who need assistance with activities of daily living. Personal care services may include help with bathing, dressing, and toileting, whereas health care services may include medication management or help with self-administration of medications. Some facilities help coordinate additional, onsite health care services such as physical and occupational therapy as well as routine medical and dental checkups.

In addition to individualized care, assisted living facilities provide three daily meals, housekeeping, exercise and wellness programs, recreational opportunities, and coordination of and/or transportation to medical, dental, and other appointments. Residents at assisted living facilities typically have their own room or living space and share common areas. Residents are typically able to bathe, dress, toilet, and eat independently or with little support. Assisted living facilities do not provide the level of skilled nursing care that is provided in nursing homes.

Nursing homes (skilled nursing facilities)

Nursing homes offer more care than assisted living facilities. In addition to many of the services offered by assisted living facilities, residents in nursing homes have access to 24-hour skilled nursing care by health care professionals and assistance with basic activities of daily living such as bathing, dressing, toileting, grooming, and eating. Nursing homes also often provide additional professional services such as physical, occupational, and respiratory therapies.

Continuing care retirement community (CCRC)

A continuing care retirement community, or CCRC, can be a good option for "aging in place." CCRCs offer a combination of independent living, assisted living, and nursing home care. Your loved one can transition through these levels of care as they are needed while still remaining on the CCRC campus. For those in independent living, services can be increased to keep your loved one independent for as long as possible before additional levels of care are needed. For example, independent living residents can choose to have all their meals provided, obtain housekeeping services, and have some personal needs cared for. In addition, healthy older adults can also live in these communities, meaning that spouses and other partners can continue to live in the same dwelling or on the same convenient campus with their loved one.

When you are evaluating a CCRC, many communities will give you the option of spending a weekend or even weeklong stay on their campus to make sure it is a good fit for you and your loved one. Keep in mind that it is important to look at all levels of the facility. In some communities the assisted living is very similar to the independent living, whereas in others moving from independent to assisted living is like moving from an apartment to a hotel room.

General housing considerations

When selecting a place for your loved one there are some general considerations you may wish to keep in mind. The first is to be sure you review the facility's admissions agreement and other contracts carefully so you understand exactly what the policies and financial commitments are for the duration of your loved one's stay. Many documents may contain legal language and a breakdown of fees that are not obvious. It can be helpful to review these documents with an attorney knowledgeable about elder law to make sure the facility policies are clear and a good fit for your loved one's needs and financial means. For CCRCs in particular, an attorney can help you determine the financial health of the facility, ensuring that the company is financially stable enough to continue offering a high level of services throughout your loved one's stay.

Second, it is best to avoid moving your loved one to another level of care in a rush or during a crisis, so you'll want to begin looking early. Most facilities have a wait list and it is sometimes many months until a spot opens up. You should also make sure you have enough time to look at several facilities to find the one that is the best fit. You may want to visit some of your top choices more than once, on different days of the week and at different times, to make sure you have the most complete view of the care your loved one will receive. The facility may also be able to provide you with names and contact information of other families with loved ones living there to serve as references.

Third, consider the location of the facility. If you are planning to visit frequently, make sure that the facility is close enough to you that you will be able to incorporate your visits into your daily, weekly, or monthly routines.

Lastly, making a move to another level of care is a big decision and one that is difficult to make alone. Recruit the help, advice, and support of family, friends, and other members of your care team during this weighty time.

Preparing for a move

Once you have made the decision to move your loved one, you may find yourself wondering how to prepare for that move. First, acknowledge that the transition may come with many emotions for everyone involved. You may experience feelings of relief, guilt, shame, loss, or anxiety. Your loved one may experience anger, fear, anxiety, depression, or disappointment. You will likely need extra support around this time.

You may need to pack up your loved one's belongings, deciding what to discard, what to move with them, what to keep elsewhere. Your loved one's space will usually be limited. Bring a few loved and memorable items, such as pictures, quilts, and bedcovers that will be comforting to your loved one and make their new surroundings feel familiar.

Making the transition

After more difficulty with incontinence and sleepless nights, Martin reluctantly agrees that Nina needs a nursing home. He and their son, James, choose one close to home so it will be easy to visit. Today they show it to her for the first time.

"So, Nina," Martin begins, "what do you think of this place? I think it's pretty nice."

Nina looks around anxiously.

A staff member comes over to them. "You must be Nina," she says, introducing herself. "We're doing an arts and crafts project right now. Would you like to join us?"

Nina looks at Martin uncertainly.

"Come on, Mama, let's go do some arts and crafts," James says as he takes her by the hand.

They leave 30 minutes later, saying, "See you tomorrow."

The next day Nina, Martin, and James sit down with some of the other residents for lunch. Martin begins to cut up Nina's chicken and sees family or staff doing the same thing for most of the residents.

After lunch, Martin says, "Let's listen to that swing music they're playing in the living room." Soon Nina is tapping her feet to the music.

"Nina, James and I need to do a couple of errands. We'll be back in a bit." He gives her a kiss and turns to go.

As they reach the door of the activity room, James asks, "Do you think Mama will be happy here, Pop?"

"I think so," Martin says, gesturing at Nina, who is swaying to the rhythm. "With a little music playing, she's completely content."

They return about 2 hours later to find her happily constructing a collage. "Why, isn't that beautiful, honey. You know, I think it's time for your nap. They've got a nice bed for you by the window."

As they make their way to Nina's room, James carries a shopping bag in each hand. He takes out a throw pillow and blanket from home and puts them on the bed. From the other bag he pulls out some framed photographs and places them on the dresser. "How's that, Mama?"

Nina lies down on the bed and Martin pulls the familiar blanket over her, just as he would do at home for her nap. He rubs her back until she falls asleep.

When she wakes up about an hour later, they have dinner in the dining room with the other residents. After dinner they take her home.

A few hours later, he lays down in bed next to her. *You know it's for the best*, he thinks, but he still cannot stop the tears as he thinks about how this is their last night together in their home.

The next day Martin and Nina arrive in time for breakfast. He stays with her the whole day.

They go to Nina's room after dinner. They talk with her roommate for a few minutes, and then Martin helps Nina get ready for bed. A staff member is present who watches, taking an occasional note on Nina's bedtime routine.

"I'll be back first thing in the morning," Martin says as he rubs her back till she falls asleep.

Martin arrives home to an empty house. He crawls into the cold bed, missing Nina terribly. He's sure he won't be able to sleep. But between the emotions of the last few days and physical exhaustion, he is soon fast asleep.

It feels like he just laid his head down when the alarm clock goes off. He the realizes that he probably hasn't had such uninterrupted sleep in several years.

Arriving at the nursing home, he's surprised to see that Nina is already up, washed, and dressed, sitting in the armchair by the window. "Are you ready to go for breakfast?" he asks as he helps her out of the chair.

Ease your loved one into the facility over a few days, as described in this story. When you are ready for their first overnight in the facility, consider making the actual move on a day when familiar staff are working, so that friendly faces who know your loved one are present. If possible, visit the next day so that your loved one understands—at least on an emotional level—that just because they are living in a new place, you are not abandoning them.

You may also choose to create a short life story or simple list of things that would help staff get to know your loved one better. You can even include photos, audio recordings, and videos if you'd like. These can include nicknames, favorite foods, music they enjoy, preferences for activities, and information about the best times of day for staff to help your loved one complete activities of daily living. You may want to include creative ways in which you have managed to get them to do something they don't like, such as bathing or taking pills. Some facilities have their own forms or guidelines to help you compile some of this useful information.

It may be difficult for you to leave your loved one on their first day in their new home. Try to make it a positive goodbye, keeping it brief and simple without a lot of emotions. If you are able to visit them the following day, remind them of that (or whenever you will next visit). Remember, you are setting the tone for your loved one.

The first few weeks may be the most difficult as your loved one adjusts to their new home. You may hear negative comments or pleas to go home. This can be difficult for you. Listening and providing the comfort of a hug or kind word can be powerful. It is important to not hastily dismiss your loved one or try to talk them out of their feelings. If they complain about a specific issue, consider it carefully. If you believe it might be warranted or have concerns of your own, don't hesitate to talk to a staff member about them.

Visiting or calling frequently for short intervals can help ease the transition. However, sometimes visits can make it more difficult for your loved one to settle in. If you or the staff notice that your visits tend to increase frustration and anger, it then makes sense to visit less frequently. It may take a couple of months for your loved one to become acclimated to their new living situation. This is an important time to turn to friends, family, or professionals for support, knowing that periods of transition are some of the most difficult parts of being a caregiver.

WHEN YOUR LOVED ONE REFUSES TO PLAN

Sometimes, despite your best efforts, your loved does not want to plan for the future. They may have always been private about their personal medical health and financial affairs and are not ready to change now. Sometimes your honest efforts to help can be seen as a threat, and they may actually believe that you are trying to steal their money. These types of paranoid feelings are not uncommon. Similarly, they may react with anger about your even mentioning the possibility of them leaving their home and going into a facility.

These situations are difficult. The first thing to mention is that it is worth bringing up these issues periodically—perhaps every few months—as people's views can change over time. It is also worthwhile to consider whether your loved one might be more receptive to hearing these issues from another member of the care team. Perhaps they would more readily accept financial help from a favorite nephew even if they are not part of the core care team. Take advantage of any strategy that works.

Do what you can unilaterally. For example, even if a bank or other financial institution cannot legally provide you with any information on your loved one's accounts or allow you to share control, you can still provide the bank with the information that you are concerned about your loved one's judgment and worry they may fall victim to scams. A bank has the right to monitor accounts for unusual activity and discuss such activity with its clients prior to releasing funds. Similarly, if your loved one is failing at home but refuses to consider appropriate facilities, you can still visit and evaluate several housing options, so that when your loved one is truly not able to live at home any longer you will be as ready as you can be.

Sometimes you may have to wait until a safety, medical, or financial crisis occurs to intervene. For example, if your loved one is admitted to the hospital or evaluated in the emergency room you can make it clear to the doctors, nurses, and social workers that you believe your loved one is no longer able to live by themselves. These providers can then work to make sure that your loved one is discharged to a setting where they will be safe. Similarly, it may take a financial crisis to occur for a judge to rule your loved one incompetent to manage their finances and give you power of attorney. Consulting with an elder law attorney can also be helpful in determining which preliminary steps you can do today.

SUMMARY

As your loved one begins to experience more problems with thinking and memory, they will need help managing their health care, finances, and other aspects of daily living. They may need to leave their home in order to receive the amount or type of care they require. Preparing legal documents such as a will, power of attorney, and health care proxy is an important step in planning for the future. Having conversations with your loved one early after a diagnosis ensures that they can participate in future planning as much as possible, easing your burden as increased care is required. Even if they don't want to participate, you can still explore options so you will be ready when a crisis occurs.

Let's consider a few examples to illustrate what we learned in this chapter.

- *You think it may be time for your loved one to move out of their home to a place that can provide them with more help, but you aren't sure. You feel overwhelmed and don't know where to start.*
  - There are several signs that may indicate it is time for a move to a facility that can provide additional care. Safety concerns, such as frequently leaving the stove on, wandering out of the house, and mismanaging medications, are signals that it may be time to consider moving your loved one out of their home. Physical aggression, violence, frequent incontinence, and other problems that make it difficult to manage your loved one at home are other indicators. Being concerned about your loved one's ability to walk safely without falling is another sign. It is always helpful to seek the advice of friends, family, and health care providers to determine whether it is the right time for a move.
- *Your father's handling of the finances in the home has always been a source of pride. Lately, however, you've noticed some delinquent payment notices in the mail and you're worried he's no longer capable of paying his bills. You'd like to ask him about these issues but are uncomfortable approaching him for fear he would become angry or depressed.*
  - Although finances may be a sensitive topic, it is critical to discuss them early—before mismanagement results in a crisis. One approach is to express your concerns to your loved one gently and ask them if they would be willing to let you watch while they manage the finances, so they can teach you what they are doing. Working together on the bills and other financial matters may be the easiest way to transition management to you when the need arises. If your loved one refuses to allow you to help and your concerns are mounting, an elder law attorney may be able to provide some assistance in determining next steps.

19

How to plan for the end and beyond

Throughout this book we have reviewed a number of topics that we hope will ease your burden and allow you to navigate caregiving to the best of your ability. This final topic, the death of your loved one, is often the most difficult one for caregivers to consider. Although death can be a sensitive topic to discuss, we believe it is important to be prepared for the passing of your loved one. We also believe it is helpful to plan for the end in the earlier stages of the disease—when your loved one can be involved in these discussions.

Some of the information that follows may be upsetting for you, such as descriptions of what to expect at the end of life. We discuss these issues because we have spoken with many caregivers who found they were ill prepared for that stage of the caregiving process and wished they had been better informed. We also want to invite you to skip this whole chapter or parts of the chapter as you see fit. We understand that not everyone is ready to consider this aspect of the caregiving experience. You are the best judge of what you wish to know now and what you would prefer to explore later.

We begin by discussing how you might initiate a conversation with your loved one about death and dying. We find the more a family understands about how their loved one wants to die, the more prepared they are when that time comes. Next, we consider aspects of the funeral ceremony they might want and how your loved one would like the setting of their death to be. We then present information about hospice and palliative care. A discussion about dying from dementia follows, including the signs that the end may be near, and whether or not to be at your loved one's side during the dying process. We note that although there may be shared features of dying from dementia, every death is unique. Next we talk about the options for the physical remains of their body, including the opportunity for your loved one to choose to donate their brain to science to help find a cure for dementia. We then discuss the grieving process and your emotional health. We end with how to plan for your own future after your loved one has died.

INVITING A CONVERSATION

"Dad, you're not dying! We don't need to talk about this now," Sara says, fighting back tears.

"I don't mean to upset you, but I don't want you guessing how I want my funeral to be," Jack says as he sees a tear escape from Sara's eye. "I want my funeral to be a celebration of my life. I want you and Claire—my daughter and granddaughter— to each tell a story. And I'd like to have a table with your first shoes, my old hockey skates, and one of Claire's soccer balls."

"Are you serious?" Sara says as she wipes the tear away.

"Why not? It's my funeral. I want people to remember what was important to me when I was alive."

That night, Sara stares at the ceiling and thinks, *I need to stop worrying about how much I'll miss him and ask him how he wants the end to be.*

The next morning Sara says, "Dad, now I know how you want your funeral to go, but what about your actual death?"

Jack takes Sara's hands in his and says, "None of us knows how the end will come. If there's time, I'd love to have you and Claire with me, holding my hands. But what's important to me is that you will both remember my stories, and Claire will pass them on to her children."

That evening at dinner Claire says, "Grandpa, Mom told me that you wanted us to pass on your stories. What about if I make a little video of you telling each of your stories? Then you can tell them to the next generation yourself."

As Jack and Claire plan the videos, Sara reflects on her journey over the last few years since her father was diagnosed with dementia.

"What are you smiling about, Mom?" Claire asks.

"Oh, I'm just enjoying listening to the two of you—the younger generation talking about how to preserve the stories of the older generation. It somehow seems right."

Yes, Sara thinks, *perhaps that's what is important in the end: focusing not how things were during the dementia, but in all of the years before.*

How does your loved one want their life to end? This is a question we encourage you to consider with them as early as possible. For some families, these conversations may come naturally, and perhaps you have already started to discuss the end of life. For others, initiating such a conversation can feel challenging or uncomfortable. Knowing what type of death your loved one wants can help you to feel more prepared when the time comes. Most families find that knowing that they are honoring their loved one's wishes at the end of life provides them with comfort and reassurance during this difficult time.

Some families find it easiest to initiate a gentle discussion with their loved one in a casual manner, a little at a time, whereas others prefer a more dedicated, serious, and extended conversation. You might start by asking your loved one if they've ever thought about the end of their life, how they imagine it would happen, and how they would like to be honored and remembered by others. Perhaps your loved one has attended a recent funeral; you may be able to use that experience to begin your conversation. Ask them what they found well done, comforting, or pleasing, and also what things they didn't like. Although these conversations may be difficult to begin and may raise emotions of sadness, grief, or fear, we find that having these conversations now will allow you, your loved one, and your family to be better prepared in the future.

THE CEREMONY

Some individuals prefer having a ceremony, whereas others would rather keep their death a more private affair. If your loved one would like a ceremony following their death, it can be helpful to discuss with them what they would like it to be and how they would like it to look. For example:

- Do they want an open or closed casket?
- Are there certain clothes they'd like to be buried in?
- Do they have a preference for a specific funeral home or religious venue?
- Would they like a ceremony and graveside service or just a ceremony alone?
- What music would they like played?
- What flowers would they like?
- Which readings should be said?
- Would they like one or more family members or friends to give a eulogy or remembrance speech?
- Is there a charity they wish to have donations sent to in lieu of flowers?

These are just a few examples of the many details that you may wish to discuss with your loved one when planning for the future.

THE DEATH ITSELF

More difficult than planning a ceremony is to consider how your loved one would like their actual death to occur. Sometimes it isn't a choice, and death comes suddenly and unexpectedly. In some circumstances, death can take time, and so it can be helpful to know what your loved one considers a "good death." A good death usually contains elements of comfort and peace. Your loved one may have a preference for where they die. Some individuals wish to die at home, whereas others prefer a hospital or hospice setting. Sometimes the exact location isn't a choice, but an individual may voice, for example, that they prefer to die near a window, with a view of the outdoors. Your loved one may wish to have family and friends around, or they may have specific requests for who they would like present and who they would prefer not to be there. They may like to have familiar things near them, such as religious or spiritual objects, a favorite blanket or shawl, or another meaningful item. Some individuals wish to have a religious figure present, such as a priest or rabbi. Other things to consider include having a certain type of music or specific song playing, and/or having flowers, particular scents, or other preferred comforts present.

CONSIDER HOSPICE AND PALLIATIVE CARE

The primary goal of hospice and palliative care is to provide a dignified death while minimizing pain. Palliative care means that treatments are aimed at comfort, not cure. Hospice care emphasizes that the remaining life expectancy is 6 months or less. In addition to providing medical care and pain management at the end of life, hospice care can also provide emotional and spiritual support, if desired, for the dying individual and their family. This care can be offered in the home or in a facility, such as a hospital, freestanding hospice center, or nursing home. Note that waiting lists for hospice care may exist, so it is helpful to start looking early. The criteria for hospice vary by facility and provider but usually include a physician's referral stating that the individual's life expectancy is 6 months or less. Make sure you fully understand the entry criteria for the hospice care you desire.

For individuals with dementia, it can be difficult to determine when 6 months of life are remaining. Experienced physicians and hospice staff can help a family determine when beginning hospice care is appropriate. It sometimes happens that an individual may begin to receive hospice care but their condition then stabilizes or improves. In these cases, the hospice care may be temporarily withdrawn and reinitiated at a later time. What usually happens in these circumstances is that the individual develops an infection—even a minor one like a cold—and their function quickly deteriorates. The decline in function may be attributed to the dementia alone, and so hospice care is initiated. When, however, the individual recovers from their infection, their function may return to its prior level.

Once you have secured hospice care, it is helpful for hospice staff to get to know your loved one. They often use forms to gather information about your loved one's spiritual beliefs, cultural background, personal preferences, nicknames, and relationships with family and friends. They may also ask about some of the topics discussed above, such as what your loved one considers a good death and their preferences for dying. You can involve your loved one in completing these forms or complete them on your own using your knowledge of them and past conversations, whichever is more appropriate under the circumstances. If your hospice provider does not have their own forms or if there is additional information you wish to communicate, you can write this information down or make it known to staff through direct conversations.

Understand hospice and palliative care

In many facilities, palliative care means that your loved one will not be transferred out for medical tests or procedures. Instead, the nurse and occasional visiting doctor will make a diagnosis just from the symptoms and bedside exam. Treatments prescribed will emphasize comfort over cure. For example, pneumonia may be treated with acetaminophen to bring the fever down and make your loved one comfortable, rather than antibiotics. Or, antibiotics may be given, but without obtaining a chest X-ray or special cultures to determine which type of pneumonia they have. Find out details from the staff exactly what palliative care means in their facility.

Hospice care also means different things in different facilities and in different hospice agencies. Sometimes it is essentially the same as palliative care plus an understanding that life expectancy is less than 6 months. However, in other facilities and agencies it indicates that your loved one is in the process of actively dying. In this latter expectation of hospice, powerful medications are used, such as morphine and other narcotics, which will provide comfort but will also cause sedation, inability to walk, and often cessation of bowel movements. When someone is actively dying, sedation, being bedridden, and cessation of bowel function are generally not important; comfort is the goal. However, if your expectation is that your loved one will live for a number of additional weeks or months, do not allow them to be given narcotics for minor discomfort or benzodiazepines for possible anxiety; these medications will hasten their death. Review these and other medication side effects in *Chapter 12*. To summarize, it is perfectly appropriate to give morphine and other powerful medications to relieve your love one's pain and discomfort when they are dying, but these are not medications that they would be able to live with for weeks or months.

DYING FROM DEMENTIA

Dementia is a fatal illness. The brain controls most parts of the body, including breathing and the regulation of the heart. For these reasons, people may die of dementia itself. However, because dementia typically begins in old age, many individuals with dementia may not reach the advanced stages and may instead die from other common causes of death, such as pneumonia, cancer, strokes, heart failure, lung disease, and complications of falls. As we have discussed in the beginning of *Step 2*, although there are a number of different types of dementia, as the dementia progresses and more of the brain becomes affected, most types of dementia produce similar problems at the end of life.

You may wonder how you will know that the end is near. Signs that the end of life might be approaching include the following:

- Needing help with most or all activities of daily living, including eating, drinking, washing, and bathing
- Eating and drinking less or not at all
- Difficulty swallowing
- Losing the ability to speak or communicate
- Losing the ability to walk or stand
- Having problems sitting up or controlling the head
- Becoming bed bound
- Constant bladder or bowel incontinence
- Recurrent infections
- Recurrent pressure ulcers or bed sores

Please note that having just one or two of these signs does not necessarily mean they will die soon. But when your loved one has many or most of these signs, it is likely that the end is near. Your loved one's health care providers should also be able to tell you when the end might be nearing, and you should feel comfortable talking with them about your questions and concerns regarding the dying process.

TO BE THERE OR NOT AT THE END

After 4 months in the nursing home, Martin has to feed Nina, and the food needs to be puréed because she doesn't chew properly. She rarely speaks. She can only walk a few steps.

Soon she spends most of her time in bed, taking in little food or drink.

"She's had a fever the last few days," Martin explains to their son, James. "They've been giving her acetaminophen suppositories to keep her comfortable. It could be any day now."

James nods and says, "Just call me."

"I will. Oh, and can you put Nina's favorite songs on my phone? She's missing her music."

"James," Martin says urgently into the phone 2 days later.

"What's wrong? Is it Mama?" James asks.

"Yes. Come quick."

Soon James is there, sitting next to his father, as Martin holds Nina's hand and strokes her hair. Nina's eyes are closed.

They are quiet, listening only to the music and Nina's occasional breaths.

"Oh, Nina," Martin says, giving her hand a squeeze, "here comes our favorite song."

> *East of the sun and west of the moon,*
> *We'll build a dream house of love, dear.*

James stands and holds her other hand gently as the music continues.

> *Up among the stars we'll find,*
> *A harmony of life to a lovely tune,*
> *East of the sun and west of the moon.*

As the song ends, Nina lets out a long noisy breath. Martin shuts off the music. Nina's body is quiet and still, undisturbed by breathing.

She looks so peaceful, Martin thinks, as he notices the sunlight streaming through the window, illuminating her face. Somehow the lines of stress and worry seem to have faded. He hears a sob, and turns to see James with tears on his face. "Come here, son," he says, and they share a long embrace.

I wonder why I'm not crying, Martin thinks.

The thought of being with your loved one at the time of their death might be frightening for you, or it may feel completely natural. Supporting a loved one through the process of dying may create an important memory for many caregivers. Being with your loved one at the time of their death or not is a personal decision. It is helpful to consider this topic early and revisit it over time, as your opinions may change throughout your loved one's disease. There may be religious, cultural, or other reasons why you and other family members may choose to be present at the time of death or not.

You should also understand that circumstances may arise that will cause you to miss this moment regardless of your choice. For example, you may have left your loved one's side for just a few minutes to get a meal and they pass while you are away. Or perhaps you receive a call that the time is near and you rush to the hospital but when you arrive they are already gone. Caregivers who wanted to be with their loved one at the time of death but couldn't be often struggle with feelings of guilt and sadness. Find peace in knowing that you did the best you could.

If you chose not to be with your loved one for other reasons, it is also important to find peace in your choice. Every person, family, and circumstance are different; there is no right way.

You may wonder what you should be doing during the dying process. You may feel uncomfortable or helpless. At this time, think of what you can do to comfort your loved one. You may have discussed some of these things when talking about their idea of a good death. You might listen to music together or sing. You can offer physical affection, such as holding your loved one's hand, stroking their hair, or giving a gentle hand massage.

This may be a time to speak with your loved one and share positive memories you have, moments of joy in your relationship. Remember that your presence alone can provide comfort to your loved one, even if it appears that they are unaware you are there.

THE BODY

You and your loved one should discuss what they wish to be done with their physical body after death. Burial is the traditional choice, either underground or above ground in a mausoleum. Burial typically involves embalming the body, allowing the funeral to take place a few days after death. Direct burial occurs without embalming, usually within one day from death, and is a less expensive option. With cremation, the remains can be scattered, kept at home, or buried in a cemetery below or above ground. Your loved one may choose to donate their organs after death to a registered organ donation and transplantation organization; see *Further Resources* for details. They may wish to donate their whole body to a medical school; contact a medical school near your loved one for more information. In each of these scenarios, individuals and their families still need to decide whether they want a ceremony to celebrate the life of their loved one and honor their death.

Consider brain donation

You or your loved one may wish to donate their brain for research. Although this is a generous contribution by itself, it is much more valuable if your loved one participates in a research program prior to death so that the doctors and scientists can learn how different brain diseases cause problems with memory, language, vision, behavior, and bodily function, and how these problems change over time. A good way to get started in the United States is to look for an Alzheimer's Disease Research Center funded by the National Institutes of Health. There are similar research programs in many other countries. See *Further Resources* for more information.

THE GRIEVING PROCESS AND YOUR EMOTIONAL HEALTH

"And so I hardly cried," Martin tells his neighbor over coffee a month after Nina's death. "I can't figure out if that's good and normal, or whether it means I have a problem."

"Well, everyone grieves differently. Most people I know cry once in a while for a year or so. But some, like you and me, did most of their mourning during the course of the dementia."

"You didn't cry much either?"

"No, I feel like I lost my father about a year before he actually died. I did most of my crying then. To be honest, when he actually died, I felt more relief than anything else. And then, of course, I felt all guilty about feeling relief."

Martin nods.

"Now, I'm no doctor," the neighbor continues, "but the way I see it, if you are functioning fine and getting on with life, I'd say you're doing OK. If, on the other hand, you're having a lot of problems, then you better go to a support group or see a therapist or something."

How do I feel? Martin thinks as he rolls over in bed. *If I'm going to be honest, I am feeling sad but also relieved. And bored. And lonely. The worst part is that when I get up in the morning, I don't know what to do with myself.*

The death of your loved one is a major transition in your journey as a caregiver. You may experience a wide range of emotions when your loved one passes, including sadness, anger, regret, relief, and guilt, to name just a few. Sometimes the death causes people to feel numb, experiencing few or no clear emotions. You may be surprised by your reactions after your loved one's death. Many caregivers feel like they've lost their loved one slowly, throughout the course of dementia (often referred to as "the long goodbye"). Others feel like they've lost their loved one twice, once when the dementia took hold and a second time when they die.

It is impossible to know exactly how you'll feel after your loved one's death. Some caregivers are more upset by the death than they expected to be, particularly if they felt there was little left of their loved one by the end and they thought they had already experienced the loss of the person. For others, the grief that occurred throughout the illness may make it easier to deal with the actual death. Reactions to the death of a loved one can vary greatly. There is no right or wrong way to grieve. It is important to be compassionate toward yourself and recognize that grief is a journey with many steps.

Working through the grief associated with your loved one's passing takes time and can be a complex process filled with various ups and downs. Find the support you need as you navigate this transition. In *Chapters 8* and *14* we suggested resources to help you cope with difficult emotions and we recommend many of those same resources at this time; see those chapters for details. Support groups specific to grieving the loss of your loved one can be helpful, as can continuing to attend your caregiver support group. Although everyone's grief is unique, support groups allow you to meet others in a similar position who may understand your feelings and may be able to offer comfort and practical suggestions for managing your grief. Individual counseling can be another place to sit with your feelings of grief and gain the support of a trained professional. You may also find comfort in those who knew your loved one—your family and friends. With your family and friends you can keep your loved one's memory alive as you process your grief together. Get the support you need. Grief does not need to be navigated alone.

PLANNING FOR YOUR FUTURE

"You can't stay in the house all the time, Pop. You can't just mourn Mama and give up living."

"You're right, son," Martin says, sighing, "but I just don't have the energy to do anything right now."

"Well, don't worry. I have enough energy for both of us. Let's start by making a list of all the people you enjoy seeing—even if you haven't seen them in ages—and the activities you like to do. Then we're going to work on scheduling them, one by one."

For the next couple of months, Martin sees friends and participates in activities that he and his son set up together.

At first, Martin feels like he is just going through the motions. Over time, however, he finds himself actually enjoying these outings.

"I still feel there's a hole in the middle," Martin says. "I'm not sad, but I just don't feel my existence has meaning now that I'm no longer caring for Nina."

"Well," his son says slowly, "a lot of things can give meaning to life."

"The one thing I keep thinking about is dementia. I'd like to help find a cure for it, so in the future people won't have to suffer like Nina did."

"That's great. Are you going to get involved in research?"

"Yes. I thought you had to have memory problems to participate in research, but they're looking for healthy older folks too."

In *Chapter 14* we introduced the concept of the "caregiver career," which starts when you begin to think of yourself as caregiver. During this time, you may be so consumed by your role that you drop many of your own interests and activities in order to focus on providing the best care. With the death of your loved one, that role comes abruptly to an end. You may be left with empty time on your hands and feel you have lost your purpose. The process of rebuilding a life for yourself after the death of your loved one is not easy—but it is vitally important.

Use the time following the death of your loved one not only to grieve but also to gradually rebuild your friendships and rediscover your hobbies and interests. Take it one step at a time. You might start by reaching out to a friend or family member for a lunch date, a cup of coffee, or a short walk. You may want to arrange a weekly meet-up with one or more friends and family members to ensure you have some time set aside each week to renew your social connections.

Make a list of all of the hobbies, activities, and interests you have had in the past as well as those you've always wanted to pursue but never had the time to. Then pick one or two of them and get started. For example, perhaps you enjoyed going to museums before your caregiving responsibilities took center stage. Now is the time to plan an outing to a museum, alone or with others, as you begin to build a life after caregiving. Perhaps you've always wanted to take a cooking class, or learn to sew, or volunteer. These types of activities can begin to fill the time you once spent providing care. Understand that the process of moving forward will take time. Some days you may not feel motivated or have the energy to take those first steps. Be patient with yourself, but stay focused on the path ahead of you.

A year after Nina's passing, Martin is finally able to stop focusing on the time when she had dementia, and instead reminisce about all the good times they shared together in their more than 60 years of marriage.

A smile creeps over his face as he looks up at the moon rising in the east among the stars.

SUMMARY

Although discussing the death of your loved one may be uncomfortable, we believe it is best to be prepared. Have conversations with your loved one about the end of their life. Consider hospice and palliative care, the death itself, the ceremony, and what should be done with their body and brain. Think about whether you wish to be present at the death. Managing grief and preparing for your future after your loved one has died are important. Find the resources you need to cope with the many emotions you may feel during the grieving process. Build a life for yourself after caregiving.

Let's consider a few examples to illustrate what we learned in this chapter.

- *My loved one and I have never discussed death. I know I should have "the conversation," but I have no idea how to broach the topic.*
  - Many people find the topic of death and dying to be uncomfortable and have trouble knowing where to begin. Talking about death doesn't have to be one long, drawn-out conversation. It can be something you talk about piece by piece in a more casual manner. You could simply tell your loved one that you'd like to better understand what their wishes are for their death, and that you can talk about it whenever they are ready.
  - It is also possible that, despite your best efforts, your loved one may not want to discuss anything related to their death. Consider what you know about them in this case and make educated guesses about how you think they'd like the end of their life to be.
- *I thought I was prepared for my loved one's death. I thought I'd be relieved that they were no longer suffering. But I find myself feeling overwhelmed and depressed. My family lives far away and I was so busy caring for my loved one that I haven't really spoken to my friends in months. I'm alone most of the time now, with nothing to do. Some days I don't even want to get out of bed. What should I do?*
  - Grief is complex and difficult. We don't always react to the loss of a loved one in the way we think we will. No one should grieve alone. Everyone needs support through the grieving process— especially when you're feeling alone, overwhelmed, and deeply saddened by your loss. Find a support group in your area where you can connect with others who are going through a similar

loss. Consider meeting with a therapist or grief counselor who can serve as a source of support. Rebuilding a life for yourself after the death of your loved one can be difficult, but it's achievable. Start with small steps. Call a friend you haven't seen in a while and go for a walk. Sign up for a class or join a gym and get yourself out of the house. The important thing is to move forward.

Glossary (with additional disorders and neuroanatomy)

Note: These definitions are accurate for how these terms pertain to memory, memory loss, dementia, and the disorders of aging discussed in this book; they are not intended to be general definitions. Neuroanatomy is also included here for those who are interested.

Alcohol-related dementia: Alcohol can cause permanent damage to the brain leading to dementia in two main ways. When intoxicated, individuals are more likely to experience head trauma that can damage the brain, due to either falling down or getting into physical fights. These trauma-related head injuries often damage the frontal lobes, leading to problems with disinhibition (see *frontal lobes*). The second way is when alcohol use is combined with nutritional deficiencies, specifically of thiamine (vitamin B1). This combination can lead to degeneration of several parts of the memory circuit (mammillary bodies and anterior nucleus of the thalamus), leading to permanent and sometimes profound amnesia. Individuals at risk for alcohol-related dementia should take thiamine daily.

Alzheimer's disease: A disorder of the brain caused by two pathologies that can be observed under a microscope, *amyloid plaques* and *neurofibrillary tangles*. Symptoms typically begin with memory loss.

Amyloid PET scan: See *PET scan*.

Amyloid plaque: Microscopic collections of beta amyloid, parts of brain cells, as well as other substances that are found between and outside brain cells. Beta amyloid is a protein that collects in *Alzheimer's disease*.

Amyotrophic lateral sclerosis (ALS): A degenerative disease that affects motor function, involving the upper and lower extremities and ultimately all muscles in the head, leading to difficulty speaking, swallowing, and breathing, and finally death. It is sometimes seen with *frontotemporal dementia*.

APOE-e4 gene: A gene that increases the probability that a person will develop *Alzheimer's disease*.

Basal ganglia: A structure deep in the center of the brain that is important for many functions, including habit or procedural learning. It is generally preserved in *Alzheimer's disease*; thus, individuals with *Alzheimer's disease* may be able to learn new habits and procedures. In *Parkinson's disease*, the basal ganglia are impaired due to a lack of dopamine, leading to slowness, stiffness, and tremor.

Cholinesterase inhibitors: Medications that improve memory by inhibiting the breakdown of the chemical acetylcholine, an important neurotransmitter in the brain. Donepezil (brand name Aricept), rivastigmine (brand name Exelon), and galantamine are three cholinesterase inhibitors commonly used to treat memory disorders and dementia, including *Alzheimer's disease, Lewy body dementia*, and *vascular dementia*.

Chronic traumatic encephalopathy (CTE): A progressive disorder of thinking, memory, mood, and behavior caused by repetitive blows to the head, such as commonly occurs in boxing and football. Note that the blows do not need to cause concussion to be damaging.

Clinical trials: Research studies of new therapies to improve cognition, behavior, or function—or to slow the decline of a brain disease. In most trials some people receive a novel medication and others receive a placebo, with the assignment being random.

Consolidation: The process by which new memories, initially formed by the hippocampus and related structures in the temporal lobe, become old memories stored in the cortex. Both rapid eye movement (REM) and non-REM sleep are important for consolidation.

Cortex: The outer layer of the brain where old consolidated memories are stored.

Corticobasal degeneration: A degenerative disease affecting thinking, memory, behavior, and movement leading to *dementia*. Different than most other dementias is that it typically begins with asymmetric involvement of an arm or a leg, leading to loss of function in that limb. The limb starts by being clumsy and progresses to becoming useless, and finally stiff and difficult to move. Some individuals experience a jerky tremor, a limb that moves seemingly with a will of its own, behavioral or personality changes, or effortful, non-fluent speech.

CT scan: A brain imaging study using X-rays that can show patterns of atrophy and *strokes*.

Dementia: When problems with thinking and memory reach the point that independent function is impaired.

Dementia with Lewy bodies: See *Lewy body dementia*.

Diabetes: Diabetes can lead to memory loss and dementia in two main ways. When blood sugar levels are not well controlled, there may be an increase in *strokes* leading to *vascular dementia*. In addition, if blood sugar levels run too low (below the normal range) it can damage the *hippocampus*, the part of the brain that forms new memories.

Distorted memory: When a memory becomes changed or mixed up with another memory such that it is no longer accurate.

False memory: When one remembers something that never happened.

Frontal lobes: Located in the front part of the brain, just behind the forehead, the frontal lobes are responsible for many cognitive and behavioral functions. The frontal lobes focus attention, allowing us to efficiently store, retrieve, and organize our memories. The left frontal lobe turns words into sounds and sentences. The frontal lobes also regulate behavior, with the inner and bottom parts inhibiting socially inappropriate responses, and the outer and top parts exploring our environment.

Frontotemporal dementia: A degenerative brain disease that affects behavior first and foremost. Typically, there are also problems related to thinking and memory, apathy or inertia, loss of sympathy or empathy, and abnormal eating behavior.

Hippocampus: The memory center of the brain, located on the inside and bottom of the temporal lobes, which are next to the temples on each side of the head, just behind the eyes. The left hippocampus is somewhat specialized for remembering verbal and factual information, and the right for nonverbal and emotional information.

Human immunodeficiency virus (HIV)–associated neurocognitive disorder (HAND): HIV disease, alone or with opportunistic infections, can cause cognitive impairment and *dementia*. Common symptoms include difficulty processing information and performing complicated tasks. Memory problems can also occur, usually due to poor learning and impaired retrieval of information.

Lewy body disease/Lewy body dementia/dementia with Lewy bodies: A degenerative brain disease that has some combination of the following symptoms: features of *Parkinson's* *disease*, visual disturbances (including hallucinations), acting-out dreams, fluctuations in attention and alertness, and thinking and memory difficulties.

Limbic-predominant age-related TDP-43 encephalopathy (LATE): A degenerative brain disease that causes symptoms similar to *Alzheimer's disease*. It is typically identified when Alzheimer's is suspected but changes in beta-amyloid protein are not observed either in an *amyloid PET scan* or in spinal fluid from a *lumbar puncture*.

Lumbar puncture: Commonly known as a spinal tap, a lumbar puncture is a procedure in which a small amount of spinal fluid is removed from the back. The fluid can be analyzed for beta *amyloid* and *tau*, two proteins whose levels are abnormal in *Alzheimer's disease*.

Mediterranean diet: One of the few diets that may be beneficial for brain health. It includes fish, vegetables, olive oil, avocados, nuts, fruits, beans, and whole grains.

Mild cognitive impairment (MCI): A term used when a decline in memory and/or thinking has been noticed and impairment is present on tests of thinking and/or memory but daily function is essentially normal, so the individual does not have *dementia*. It is a pre-dementia stage. Individuals may have mild cognitive impairment due to *Alzheimer's disease*, cerebrovascular disease, *Lewy body disease*, or another disorder. (For more information, see our book *Seven Steps to Managing Your Memory*.)

MRI scan: A brain imaging study using powerful magnets that can show patterns of atrophy and *strokes*.

Multiple sclerosis (as a cause of *dementia*): A disease of the brain and spinal cord in which the myelin—the insulation around nerves—is disrupted by an autoimmune process. It typically presents with noticeable symptoms over hours or days, which may or may not resolve. Many individuals with multiple sclerosis never develop cognitive problems or dementia. When dementia does appear, it typically presents with slowed processing, inability to perform complicated activities, and easy or abnormal laughing and crying (*pseudobulbar affect*).

Neurofibrillary tangle: Parts of the skeleton and nutrient system of the dying brain cell that appear "tangled" under the microscope. These tangles, made up of *tau*, form after the cell has been damaged by *amyloid plaques* or another process.

Neurological exam: A specialized physical exam to evaluate the brain and nervous system. It includes testing vision, hearing, strength, sensation, movement, walking, and reflexes.

Neurologist: A medical doctor who specializes in the diagnosis and treatment of disorders of the brain and other parts of the nervous system.

Neuropsychological examination: A comprehensive interview along with questionnaires and pencil-and-paper or computerized tests to evaluate different aspects of thinking, memory, mood, and behavior in order to determine how different parts of the brain are functioning. Results are used to guide diagnosis and treatment.

Neuropsychologist: A psychologist who has received advanced training in the use and interpretation of pencil-and-paper and computerized tests and questionnaires to help diagnose brain disorders and provide practical advice.

Normal pressure hydrocephalus: A disorder caused by excess fluid in the brain, leading to slowing of walking with small steps; urgency to run to the bathroom to urinate; and poor attention, thinking, and memory.

Occipital lobes: The back, lower parts of the brain where visual perception takes place. The eye turns images (of a dog, for example) into neural impulses that travel through nerves to your occipital lobes in the back of your brain. The left occipital lobe recreates the images on the right side of your vision (the dog's head, for example, if it is facing to the right), and the right occipital lobe recreates the images on the left side of your vision (the dog's body, for example). Once the image of the dog has been recreated by the occipital lobe, the image is transferred to the *temporal* and *parietal lobes*.

Parietal lobes: The back, upper parts of the brain that are important for attention and spatial functioning; they are affected early in the course of *Alzheimer's disease*, *Lewy body dementia*, and *posterior cortical atrophy*. If an image of a dog reaches your parietal lobes, you will know where the dog is; what direction it is facing; and whether it is walking, running, or standing still. The parietal lobes also help to pay attention. Here parietal lobe function is asymmetric: The right parietal lobe can pay attention to either the left or right side, whereas the left parietal lobe only pays attention to the right. This asymmetry means that if there is damage to the left parietal lobe, attention can still be paid to both sides, but when there is damage to the right parietal lobe, attention cannot be paid to the left side, and things on the left are neglected.

Parkinson's disease: A degenerative brain disease causing some combination of slowness of movement; slow, shuffling walking; and a tremor. Other symptoms can include loss of smell, constipation, and REM sleep behavior disorder. It may be treated by medications.

PET scan: A positron emission tomography (PET) scan is like an "inside-out" X-ray. With an X-ray, the radiation beams go from the transmitter through the body and then collect on a film or X-ray detector. With an *amyloid* or *tau* PET scan, the radiation is built into a tiny molecule that is engineered to stick to either amyloid plaques or tau tangles. The molecule is injected through an intravenous (IV) catheter in the arm, and if there are any amyloid plaques or tau tangles in the brain it will stick to them. The radiation of the molecule sticking to the plaques or tangles is then detected on the X-ray detector.

***Posterior cortical atrophy*:** Although not a disease in itself, this term is a useful way to describe individuals with *dementia* who have visual problems as their most prominent symptom, while their other cognitive functions (such as memory, language, and behavior) are more or less intact. The name comes from the fact that the back or posterior part of the brain is most affected.

***Primary age-related tauopathy (PART)*:** A degenerative disease in which *tau neurofibrillary tangles* develop in the *temporal lobes*, leading to slowness of cognition and difficulty performing complicated tasks. It is not thought to lead to *dementia*.

***Primary progressive aphasia*:** A degenerative brain disorder that affects language first and foremost.

***Progressive supranuclear palsy (PSP)*:** A degenerative brain disease affecting thinking, memory, behavior, function, balance, speech, and eye movements. Individuals often begin with a slowing of eye movements and difficulty walking due to poor balance. They typically progress to difficulty looking down, frequent falls, speech difficulties, and swallowing problems, in addition to impairment in thinking, memory, and behavior.

***Pseudobulbar affect*:** A disorder common in *dementia* in which individuals may laugh or cry with little or no provocation. Treatment is available.

***Rapid forgetting*:** Even when information has been learned well, it is quickly forgotten, often leading to repeating questions and leaving important items unattended, such as leaving the stove on.

***Stroke*:** Occurs when an artery sending blood from the heart to the brain becomes blocked off; that part of the brain doesn't receive enough blood and dies. Because the problem is related to blood vessels, strokes are often called "vascular disease" or sometimes "cerebrovascular disease" to emphasize that the problem is with blood vessels of the brain or "cerebrum." Small-vessel disease strokes from the blockage of small and microscopic arteries in the brain are typically silent and only detected on *CT* or *MRI scans*.

Subjective cognitive decline: A term used when a decline in thinking and/or memory has been noticed by the individual, and it is of sufficient concern to bring it to the attention of a doctor, but tests of thinking and memory are normal, as is daily function. (For more information, see our book *Seven Steps to Managing Your Memory*.)

Tau: A protein that is part of the skeleton and nutrient system of the brain cells. See also *neurofibrillary tangle*.

Tau PET scan: See *PET scan*.

Temporal lobes: The temporal lobes tell you what you are looking at and your emotional connection to it, in addition to storing your vocabulary. If an image of a dog reaches your temporal lobes, you will be able to identify the image as a dog, what color its hair is, and which breed it is. The left temporal lobe contains your vocabulary, turning meaning into words. In each temporal lobe are the emotional centers of the brain, almond-shaped structures called amygdala. When the image reaches the amygdala, it produces the appropriate emotion: affection if it is your dog and wariness if you have never seen the dog before.

Thyroid: A gland in the neck that produces thyroid hormone. Abnormal thyroid hormone levels may cause impaired memory, difficulty concentrating, irritability, mood instability, restlessness, and confusion.

Vascular cognitive impairment: *Cognitive impairment* due to *strokes*.

Vascular dementia: *Dementia* due to *strokes*.

Vitamin B12: Deficiency of vitamin B12 can cause serious problems with thinking, memory, and mood. Some individuals require B12 injections as they are unable to absorb B12 even if their dietary intake is normal.

Vitamin D: Deficiency of vitamin D has been associated with a higher risk of *dementia* in general and *Alzheimer's disease* in particular.

Further resources

ADULT DAY CENTERS

The Alzheimer's Association has a helpful printout listing the types of questions you may want to ask when exploring adult day centers for your loved one: www.alz.org/national/documents/topicsheet_adultday.pdf.

ALZHEIMER'S DISEASE RESEARCH CENTERS

There are more than 30 Alzheimer's Disease Research Centers funded by the National Institutes of Health (www.nia.nih.gov/health/alzheimers-disease-research-centers). Although focused primarily on research, these centers also provide resources for the community. Contact one close to you to find out more information. There are similar research programs in many other countries.

COMPANIONSHIP AND ASSISTANCE

Senior Corps is an organization that has senior volunteers who can provide companionship and assistance to older adults with dementia (www.nationalservice.gov/programs/senior-corps).

DRIVING

These two links provide helpful information regarding driving and dementia: https://www.thehartford.com/resources/mature-market-excellence/publications-on-aging http://www.alz.org/care/alzheimers-dementia-and-driving.asp.

EXERCISE

Silver Sneakers is a program that provides seniors with free access to fitness equipment and classes at over 14,000 locations nationally and can be a resource for finding fitness classes (www.silversneakers.com).

GERIATRIC CARE MANAGERS

The Aging Life Care Association (www.aginglifecare.org; formerly the National Association of Professional Geriatric Care Managers) will help you get connected with a geriatric care manager in your area.

IDENTIFICATION BRACELETS

The most commonly used system is the MedicAlert® + Alzheimer's Association Safe Return® 24-hour nationwide emergency response service (https://www.alz.org/help-support/caregiving/safety/medicalert-safe-return). The system costs less than $75 to set up and can be joined by calling 888-572-8566 or going to www.medicalert.org/safereturn.

MEDICAL STUDENT PROGRAMS

A number of medical schools across the United Sates pair individuals with Alzheimer's disease with medical students to cultivate a relationships that helps these young medical professionals improve their knowledge of dementia and the lived experience of having dementia, improve their communication skills with individuals with dementia, and foster enthusiasm for career opportunities in neurology, psychiatry, and geriatrics. Contact a medical school near you if you are interested.

MEDICATION TRACKING

You can use this link from the National Institute on Aging to track your loved one's medications (https://www.nia.nih.gov/health/tracking-your-medications-worksheet).

MEDITATION

You can use this link from the National Institutes of Health to learn more about meditation (https://nccih.nih.gov/health/meditation/overview.htm).

ORGAN DONATION

Information about organ donation and transplantation can be found at www.organdonor.gov.

ORGANIZATIONS

Many countries have national organizations dedicated to helping people with Alzheimer's disease and other causes of dementia and their caregivers. In addition to informational websites, online support groups, and telephone help lines, these organizations typically have local chapters offering numerous resources that may be in or near your community. Look for the Alzheimer's Association in the United States (www.alz.org; 800-272-3900) and Australia (https://www.alz.org/au/dementia-alzheimers-australia.asp), Alzheimer Society in Canada (https://alzheimer.ca/en; 800-616-8816), and Alzheimer's Society throughout much of the United Kingdom (www.alzheimers.org.uk; 0300 222 1122). Your local community center and faith-based groups may also offer resources for you and your loved one with dementia.

RELAXATION THERAPY

You can use this link from the National Institutes of Health to learn more about relaxation therapy (https://nccih.nih.gov/health/stress/relaxation.htm).

RESPITE CARE

Financial assistance for respite care may be available through federal, state, or local organizations, such as the National Family Caregiver Support Program (information can be found at www.payingforseniorcare.com) and the Lifespan Respite Care Program (https://archrespite.org/lifespan-programs).

SHARED CALENDARS

Lotsa Helping Hands (www.lotsahelpinghands.com), Caring Bridge (https://www.caringbridge.org), and Caring Village (www.caringvillage.com).

SUPPORT GROUPS

The Alzheimer's Association in the United States hosts a number of online support groups and classes via platforms such as www.ALZconnected.org, a free online caregiver support community, and their community resource finder that includes free online classes to teach caregivers things like how to communicate better with a loved one with dementia and get legal and financial affairs in order following a diagnosis of dementia. Other countries have similar programs. Many medical centers and clinics and some religious organizations also offer support groups.

About the authors

Andrew E. Budson received his bachelor's degree at Haverford College where he majored in both chemistry and philosophy. After graduating *cum laude* from Harvard Medical School, he was an intern in internal medicine at Brigham and Women's Hospital. He then attended the Harvard-Longwood Neurology Residency Program, for which he was chosen to be chief resident in his senior year. He next pursued a fellowship in behavioral neurology and dementia at Brigham and Women's Hospital, after which he joined the neurology department there. He participated in numerous clinical trials of new drugs to treat Alzheimer's disease in his role as the Associate Medical Director of Clinical Trials for Alzheimer's Disease at Brigham and Women's Hospital. Following his clinical training he spent three years studying memory as a post-doctoral fellow in experimental psychology and cognitive neuroscience at Harvard University under Professor Daniel Schacter. After 5 years as Assistant Professor of Neurology at Harvard Medical School, he joined the Boston University Alzheimer's Disease Research Center and the Geriatric Research Education Clinical Center (GRECC) at the Bedford Veterans Affairs Hospital. During his 5 years at the Bedford GRECC he served in several roles including the Director of Outpatient Services, Associate Clinical Director, and later the overall GRECC Director. In 2010 he moved to the Veterans Affairs Boston Healthcare System, where he is currently the Associate Chief of Staff for Education, Chief of Cognitive & Behavioral Neurology, and Director of the Center for Translational Cognitive Neuroscience. He is also the Director of Outreach, Recruitment, and Education at the Boston University Alzheimer's Disease Research Center, Professor of Neurology at Boston University School of Medicine, and Lecturer in Neurology at Harvard Medical School. Dr. Budson has had National Institutes of Health and other government research funding since 1998, receiving a National Research Service Award and a Career Development Award in addition to Research Project (R01) and VA Merit grants. He has given over 650 local, national, and international grand rounds and other academic talks, including at the Institute of Cognitive Neuroscience, Queen Square, London; Berlin, Germany; and Cambridge University, England. He has published over 100 papers in peer-reviewed journals, including *The New England Journal of Medicine, Brain,* and *Cortex,* and is a reviewer for more than 50 journals. He was awarded the Norman Geschwind Prize in Behavioral Neurology in 2008 and the Research Award in Geriatric Neurology in 2009, both from the American Academy of Neurology. His current research uses the techniques of experimental psychology and cognitive neuroscience to understand memory and memory distortions in patients with Alzheimer's disease and other neurological disorders. In his Memory Disorders Clinic at the Veterans Affairs Boston Healthcare System he treats patients while teaching medical students, residents, and fellows. He also sees patients at the Boston Center for Memory in Newton, Massachusetts. When not working or writing, he enjoys spending time with his family, traveling, running, skiing, and biking.

Maureen K . O'Connor graduated *summa cum laude* with a bachelor's degree from Ithaca College, where she majored in both psychology and religion. She received her doctorate in psychology from Indiana University of Pennsylvania, focusing her dissertation on the differentiation of depression versus Alzheimer's disease under the mentorship of Dr. David LaPorte. She attended Yale University School of Medicine for her predoctoral internship, where she conducted outpatient and inpatient memory evaluations for adults with a broad range of diagnostic presentations, including dementia, traumatic brain injury, and stroke. She went on to complete 1 year of postdoctoral residency at Cornell Weil Medical Center/Sloan Kettering Cancer Center and 2 additional years of residency at the Bedford

Veterans Affairs Hospital/Boston University School of Medicine. In 2005 she accepted an appointment at the Bedford Veterans Affairs Hospital as the Director of Neuropsychology. In that role she established the Memory Diagnostic Clinic, specifically designed to evaluate and treat older Veterans with memory loss. In 2008 she was awarded board certification in neuropsychology by the American Board of Professional Psychology. In 2009 she accepted the Young Alumni Achievement Award from the College of Natural Sciences and Mathematics at Indiana University of Pennsylvania. She has served on the board of the Massachusetts Neuropsychological Society as the Chair of the Continuing Education Committee and on the board of the National Academy of Neuropsychology as the Chair of the Education Committee and Member at Large. In 2014 she was promoted to the rank of Assistant Professor in the Department of Neurology at Boston University School of Medicine. She has served as the Associate Director of the Outreach, Recruitment, and Education Core at the Boston University Alzheimer's Disease Center and is the current Director of the Research Education Component. Dr. O'Connor's research interests include understanding and developing interventions to improve the lives of adults with memory loss and the lives of the family members who help provide care. In 2005 she received a pilot grant from the Boston University Alzheimer's Disease Center to study the effect of exercise training on cognition. In 2006 she was the recipient of a New Investigator Research Grant from the National Alzheimer's Association designed to study the impact of caregiver training on managing neuropsychiatric symptoms in dementia. In 2014 she was awarded a Research, Rehabilitation, and Development SPiRE Award to study the impact of an intervention designed to educate older adults about brain aging and dementia and lifestyle factors that contribute to brain aging. Her recent funding from the National Institute on Aging (NIA) supports research designed to understand how couples' relationships change over the course of navigating a diagnosis of dementia and contribute to disease outcomes. In addition to her research, Dr. O'Connor continues to evaluate and treat individuals with memory loss while teaching doctoral students, interns, and residents in neuropsychology. In her free time she enjoys running, cooking, and relaxing with her husband and daughter, and the family dog, Bruce.

Index

For the benefit of digital users, indexed terms that span two pages (e.g., 52–53) may, on occasion, appear on only one of those pages.

Tables are indicated by *t* following the page number

Index